Wicke · Atlas of Radiologic Anatomy

Third Edition

# Atlas of Radiologic Anatomy

By Lothar Wicke

With the Assistance of
Wilhelm Firbas and Roland Schmiedl

Radiographs by
Heinrich Brenner, Wilfried Czech, Erich Deimer, Hans Heeger,
Ernst Kotscher, Emanuele Maranta, Friedrich Olbert,
Axel Perneczky, Peter Probst, Thomas Reisner, Wolfgang Schwägerl,
Christl Wicke, Lothar Wicke and Georg Wolf

Third Edition

128 Radiographs and 128 Line Drawings

Urban & Schwarzenberg · Baltimore–Munich 1982

Urban & Schwarzenberg. Inc.
7 East Redwood Street
Baltimore, Maryland 21 202 U.S.A.

Urban & Schwarzenberg
Pettenkoferstrasse 18
D-8000 Munich 2
Germany

© 1982 by Urban & Schwarzenberg

Translated by Allan L. Rice, Ph.D.
With editorial assistance from:
Michael Dooley, M.D.
Allan Cohen, M.D.
Klemens H. Barth, M.D.

Translating and editing of the
figure labels by:
Dallas R. Boushey
Patricia P. Krupp, Ph.D.

A translation of
Atlas der Röntgenanatomie, Urban & Schwarzenberg, München 1980

**Library of Congress Cataloging in Publication Data**

Wicke, Lothar.
  Atlas of radiologic anatomy.

  Translation of Atlas der Röntgenanatomie.
  Includes index.
  1. Diagnosis, Radioscopic--Atlases.  2. Anatomy,
Human--Atlases.  I. Firbas, Wilhelm.  II. Schmiedl,
Roland.  III.  Title. [DNLM: 1. Anatomy--Atlases.
2. Radiography--Atlases.  WN 17 W636a]
RC78.2.W5313  1982      611'.0022'2      81-23977
ISBN 0-8067-2113-8             AACR2

Printed in Germany

ISBN 0-8067-2113-8 Baltimore

ISBN 3-541-72113-8 München

# Foreword

The authors of this book have set out to perpetuate the long tradition of anatomic-radiologic correlation at the University of Vienna, Institute of Anatomy.

The extensive atlas, with more than 100 carefully selected radiographs, systematically arranged and unmarred by intrusive lines or markings, is eminently suited for the study of anatomic details and is enhanced by explanatory line drawings of the radiographs. The selection includes not only skeletal radiography of limited special areas, but covers the essential aspects of roentgen anatomy in all parts of the body.

Careful editing and, not least, the format and moderate price should allow this book a wide circulation.

Vienna, 1981

H. Ferner, M.D.
Professor of Anatomy
University of Vienna

# Preface to the Third Edition

The wide acceptance and use of previous editions of this book have been a direct result of the quality of its illustrations; we have not, therefore, changed their basic selection. However, in response to the many suggestions received from readers and reviewers, many radiographs have been rephotographed and now have even more contrast and clarity of focus. The most significant change in this new edition is the reversal from positive to negative printing of the radiographs. This has been done so that the radiographs will appear in a format identical to that most frequently seen in clinical practice.

It is our hope that this book will continue to be used as a basic reference in radiologic anatomy by medical students, students of radiologic technology, and radiologists-in-training, as well as by those practicing physicians who wish to increase their understanding of radiologic correlative anatomy.

Special thanks are given to Urban & Schwarzenberg, who generously considered our wishes, and who again have produced a book of excellent quality.

Vienna, 1981                    Lothar Wicke, M.D., F.I.C.A.

# Preface to the First Edition

The ever-increasing inclusion of radiologic diagnosis in anatomic instruction and clinical training has prompted the organization of this volume. It affords the student an opportunity to check an expand his knowledge of the anatomic details that are observable by radiology, with guidance from the sketches accompanying each radiograph.

The illustrations have been selected under the aspect of the broadest possible basic coverage of radiologic anatomy. In our opinion they include all common roentgen examinations with which students, technicians and house staff may be confronted. We have intentionally dispensed with many specialized exposure and projection techniques which would have expanded the intended scope of the book and which are readily accessible in more specialized works to all those interested.

We are deeply obligated to our professor in anatomy, Dr. W. Krause, for his generous critical supervision of the captions and labeling of all the illustrations in the atlas. We are also grateful to the publishers for their care in achieving optimal reproduction of the radiographs and line drawings. The original radiographs were electronically contrast enhanced and converted into positives for use in the book, since only in this form do we feel the best detail is to be captured. The disadvantage, namely that the radiographs do not appear as negatives, the way radiologists see them in practice, is outweighed in our opinion by the picture quality. As for terminology, we used the Wiesbaden anatomic nomenclature of 1965, as often as suitable terms were available. Special designations which are only in clinical or radiologic use are marked with an asterisk (*).

It is our hope that we will have made available in this atlas a practical ready-reference guide for those interested in acquiring the basic knowledge of radiologic anatomy as applied to clinical radiology.

Vienna, December 1977

Lothar Wicke, M.D., F.I.C.A.

Wilhelm Firbas, M.D.

Roland Schmiedl, M.D.

# Preface to the Second Edition

The success of the first edition of this atlas has prompted the publication of a revision in just 18 months. In order to make the book more useful to students in North America, English nomenclature has been used throughout. The kind assistance of Dallas R. Boushey and Patricia P. Krupp of the Department of Anatomy, University of Vermont College of Medicine, in translating and editing the figure labels is gratefully acknowledged.

St. Pölten, March 1979

L. Wicke, M.D., F.I.C.A.
Chief of Radiologic Institute,
Allgemeines Öffentliches Krankenhaus,
St. Pölten – Austria

# Table of Contents

Foreword . . . . . . . . . . . . . . . . . . . . . . . . . . . . . . v

Prefaces . . . . . . . . . . . . . . . . . . . . . . . . . . . . . . v

Atlas . . . . . . . . . . . . . . . . . . . . . . . . . . . . . . . . 1

## Skull
Skull (p.a., lateral, axial projections) . . . . . . . . . . . 2
Paranasal sinuses (p.a., Water's, axial projections) . . 10
Orbitae (p.a. projection) . . . . . . . . . . . . . . . . . . . . . 12
Canalis opticus (after Rhese) . . . . . . . . . . . . . . . 14
Temporal bone (semisagittal, Stenvers; semilateral,
    Schüller; semiaxial projections, Mayer) . . . . . . . 14
Upper and lower jaws (panoramic projections) . . . 18
Carotid angiography (lateral, a.p. projections,
    venous phases) . . . . . . . . . . . . . . . . . . . . . . . . 20
Vertebral angiography (lateral, a.p. projections,
    venous phase) . . . . . . . . . . . . . . . . . . . . . . . . 32
Ventriculography (a.p., lateral projections;
    Pantopaque ventriculogram) . . . . . . . . . . . . . . 38
Sella turcica (coned-down projection) . . . . . . . . . 42

## Spinal Column
Cervical spine (a.p., lateral projections;
    odontoid bone in a.p. projection) . . . . . . . . . . . 44
Cervical spine (functional exposures) . . . . . . . . . . 50
Cervical spine (antero-oblique projection) . . . . . . . 54
Thoracic spine (a.p., lateral projections) . . . . . . . . 56
Lumbar spine (a.p., lateral, oblique projections) . . 58
Myelography (p.a., lateral projections) . . . . . . . . 64

## Pelvis
Pelvis (a.p., lateral projections) . . . . . . . . . . . . . 68
Sacrum (lateral projection) . . . . . . . . . . . . . . . . . 70
Iliac arteries . . . . . . . . . . . . . . . . . . . . . . . . . . . 72

## Upper Extremity
Shoulder (a.p., axial projections) . . . . . . . . . . . . . 74
Elbow (a.p., lateral projections; arteriogram) . . . . 78

Hand (dorsovolar, lateral, latero-oblique
    projections; arteriogram) . . . . . . . . . . . . . . . . . 82

## Lower Extremity
Hip joint (a.p., lateral projection with leg laterally
    abducted (Lauenstein) . . . . . . . . . . . . . . . . . . 90
Child's hip joint . . . . . . . . . . . . . . . . . . . . . . . . 94
Knee joint (a.p., lateral projections;
    lateral arthrogram) . . . . . . . . . . . . . . . . . . . . . 96
Patella (axial projection) . . . . . . . . . . . . . . . . . . 102
Knee joint, arthrography; arteriogram
    (a.p. projections) . . . . . . . . . . . . . . . . . . . . . . 102
Ankle joint (a.p., lateral, oblique projections) . . . . 106
Foot (dorsoplantar, lateral projections) . . . . . . . . 110
Ankle joint, angiography (a.p. projection) . . . . . . . 114

## Thorax and Neck
Lungs (p.a., lateral projections) . . . . . . . . . . . . . 116
Lung tomography (a.p. projection) . . . . . . . . . . . 120
Right bronchography (a.p., steep oblique
    projections) . . . . . . . . . . . . . . . . . . . . . . . . . . 122
Left bronchography (a.p., steep oblique
    projections) . . . . . . . . . . . . . . . . . . . . . . . . . . 126
Mediastinography (lateral tomogram) . . . . . . . . . 130
Heart (p.a., right and left
    antero-oblique projections) . . . . . . . . . . . . . . . 132
Venous angiocardiography . . . . . . . . . . . . . . . . . 138
Levo phase . . . . . . . . . . . . . . . . . . . . . . . . . . . 140
Aortic arch . . . . . . . . . . . . . . . . . . . . . . . . . . . 142
Right coronary artery (left antero-oblique,
    lateral projections) . . . . . . . . . . . . . . . . . . . . . 144
Left coronary artery (right and left
    antero-oblique projections) . . . . . . . . . . . . . . . 148
Mammography (cranio-caudal, lateral
    projections) . . . . . . . . . . . . . . . . . . . . . . . . . . 152
Trachea (a. p., lateral projections) . . . . . . . . . . . . 156

## Digestive Tract
Hypopharynx (p.a., lateral projections) . . . . . . . . 160
Esophagus (right and left antero-
    oblique projections) . . . . . . . . . . . . . . . . . . . . 164

Stomach (p.a. projections; patient erect, reclining) . 166
Duodenum (right antero-oblique projection) . . . . . 172
Jejunum and ileum . . . . . . . . . . . . . . . . . . . . . . 174
Celiac arteriography . . . . . . . . . . . . . . . . . . . . . 176
Indirect splenoportography . . . . . . . . . . . . . . . . 178
Superior mesenteric arteriography . . . . . . . . . . . 180
Inferior mesenteric arteriography . . . . . . . . . . . 182
Colon (fully filled, post-evacuation, irrigoradio-
    scopy, double contrast) . . . . . . . . . . . . . . . . . 184

**Biliary Tract**
Gall bladder (oral cholecystography before and
    after fatty meal) . . . . . . . . . . . . . . . . . . . . . . 192
Intravenous cholangiography . . . . . . . . . . . . . . . 196
Retrograde cholangiography . . . . . . . . . . . . . . . 198
Intraoperative cholangiography . . . . . . . . . . . . . 200

**Kidneys and Urinary Tract**
Intravenous urography . . . . . . . . . . . . . . . . . . . 202
Intravenous urography (section
    through left kidney) . . . . . . . . . . . . . . . . . . . 204
Selective renal arteriography . . . . . . . . . . . . . . . 204

Abdominal aortography . . . . . . . . . . . . . . . . . . . 206
Retroperitoneal air study (tomogram) . . . . . . . . . 208

**Veins**
Phlebography of lower extremity
    (p.a., lateral projections) . . . . . . . . . . . . . . . . 210
Venous valve . . . . . . . . . . . . . . . . . . . . . . . . . . 212

**Lymphatic System**
Pelvis and para-aortic region, nodal phase
    (a.p., lateral, oblique projections) . . . . . . . . . . 214
Inguinal lymph nodes (vascular phase) . . . . . . . . 222
Axillary lymph nodes (nodal phase) . . . . . . . . . . 224
Thoracic duct . . . . . . . . . . . . . . . . . . . . . . . . . 226

**Gynecologic Radiography**
Hysterosalpingography . . . . . . . . . . . . . . . . . . . 228
Fetography . . . . . . . . . . . . . . . . . . . . . . . . . . . 230

Bibliography . . . . . . . . . . . . . . . . . . . . . . . . . . 232

Subject index . . . . . . . . . . . . . . . . . . . . . . . . . 233

# Atlas

The figures in the atlas are negative copies of original x-ray films of a living person, except the view which is from the skeleton skull (Fig. 5) without mandibles.

In roentgenology, the directions are specified in a way that always the particular direction is shown where the central ray passes through the patient from the x-ray tube to the cassette resp. screen. The x-ray pictures are observed correspondingly, as if the patient were standing right in front of the examiner. There are only few exceptions of this rule in practice (e.g. hand dorsovolar, front foot dorsoplantar).

Lead marks are frequently shown on the x-ray film for the identification of the respective body half (R for right, L for left).

Periodic scales were added for pictures which are taken in certain time intervalls after the final injection (e.g. urograms). In order to carry out an exact localisation in the body, pictures are frequently taken in another ray passage, besides sectional roentgenography. Thus pictures of the skull are taken in the posterior–anterior and in the lateral (= frontal) ray passage; when x-raying the stomach, or expecially taking x-rays at cardiac diagnostics, it is recommended to carry out the fluoroscopy and the pictures in the anterior oblique projections. The most important directional specifications are listed below for further information (Fig. 1).

(1)   p.a.: posterior anterior (in this case in the median-sagittal-plane);
(2)   lateral: from the side;
(3)   frontal: parallel to the front plane;
(4)   right anterior oblique projection (position of a fencer); the patient is turned around his axis in a way that the x-rays pass through him from the left back to the right front;
(5)   left anterior ablique projection (position of a boxer); the patient is turned around his axis in a way that the x-rays pass through him from the right back to the left front;
(6)   sagittal: parallel to the median plane (p.a.or a.p.);

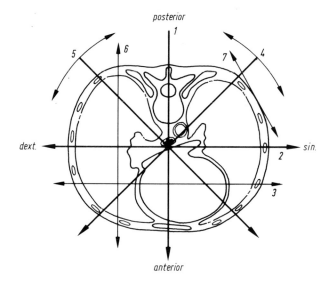

Fig. 1.  Frequent directional identifications.

(7)   tangential: the central ray is tangent to a bended surface in one point.
a.p.:   anterior posterior;
ds:   from right (dexter) to left (sinister);
sd:   rom left (sinister) to right (dexter);
dv:   (concerning the hand) = dorsovolar: from the back of the hand to its palm;
dp:   dorsoplantar: from the back of the foot to its sole;
radio-ulnar: from the radius to the ulna;
axial: in the direction of the longitudinal axis of the body when standing upright.

Besides, the anatomic specifications like cranial, caudal, proximal, distal, dorsal, ventral, transversal, are valid.

There are outlines in order to simplify the imagination of how the x-ray pictures were taken.

The central ray of the x-ray bundle was marked with an arrow in its direction, the film cassette is shown by a thick line.

The orbitomental line (connecting line between the lower margin of the orbita and the upper limitation of the outer auditory passage) is drawn with a dash-dot-dash line (_._._).

# Skull

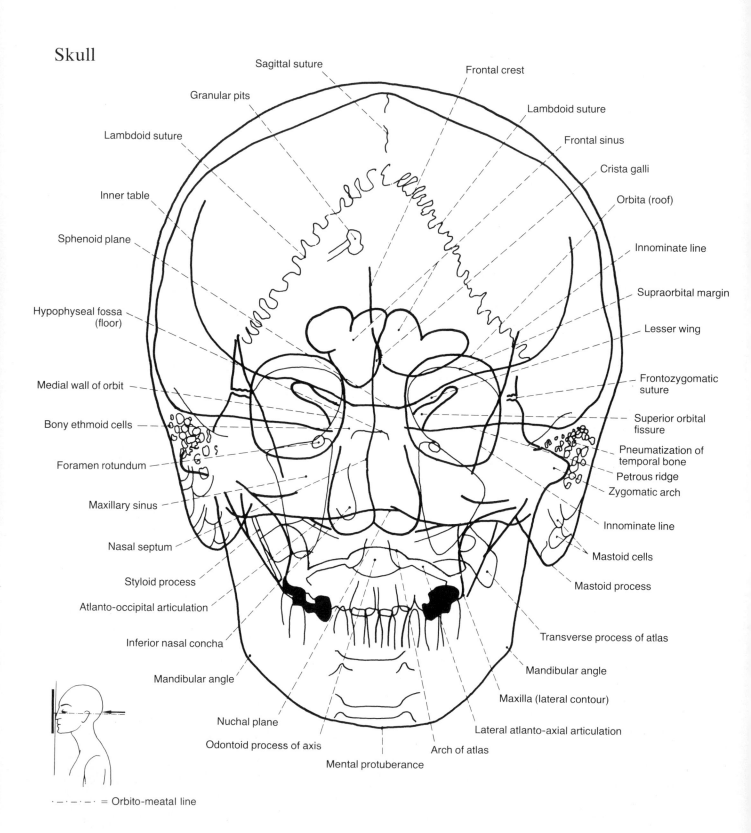

Sagittal suture

Frontal crest

Granular pits

Lambdoid suture

Lambdoid suture

Frontal sinus

Inner table

Crista galli

Sphenoid plane

Orbita (roof)

Innominate line

Hypophyseal fossa (floor)

Supraorbital margin

Lesser wing

Medial wall of orbit

Frontozygomatic suture

Bony ethmoid cells

Superior orbital fissure

Foramen rotundum

Pneumatization of temporal bone

Petrous ridge

Maxillary sinus

Zygomatic arch

Nasal septum

Innominate line

Styloid process

Mastoid cells

Atlanto-occipital articulation

Mastoid process

Inferior nasal concha

Transverse process of atlas

Mandibular angle

Mandibular angle

Maxilla (lateral contour)

Nuchal plane

Lateral atlanto-axial articulation

Odontoid process of axis

Arch of atlas

Mental protuberance

$-\cdot-\cdot-\cdot-$ = Orbito-meatal line

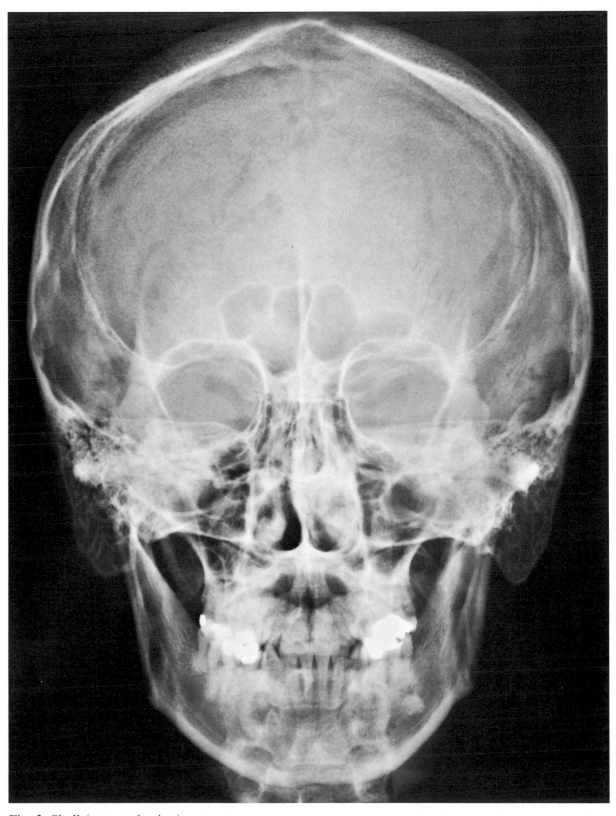

Fig. 2. Skull (p.a. projection)

# Skull

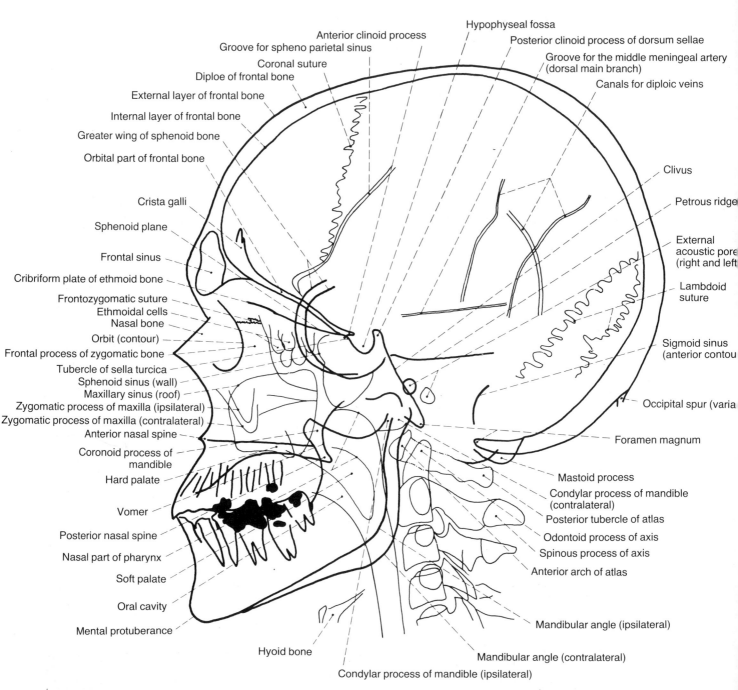

Hypophyseal fossa

Anterior clinoid process

Posterior clinoid process of dorsum sellae

Groove for spheno parietal sinus

Groove for the middle meningeal artery
(dorsal main branch)

Coronal suture

Canals for diploic veins

Diploe of frontal bone

External layer of frontal bone

Internal layer of frontal bone

Greater wing of sphenoid bone

Orbital part of frontal bone

Clivus

Petrous ridge

Crista galli

Sphenoid plane

External
acoustic pore
(right and left)

Frontal sinus

Cribriform plate of ethmoid bone

Lambdoid
suture

Frontozygomatic suture

Ethmoidal cells

Nasal bone

Sigmoid sinus
(anterior contour)

Orbit (contour)

Frontal process of zygomatic bone

Tubercle of sella turcica

Sphenoid sinus (wall)

Maxillary sinus (roof)

Zygomatic process of maxilla (ipsilateral)

Occipital spur (varia)

Zygomatic process of maxilla (contralateral)

Anterior nasal spine

Foramen magnum

Coronoid process of
mandible

Hard palate

Mastoid process

Condylar process of mandible
(contralateral)

Vomer

Posterior tubercle of atlas

Posterior nasal spine

Odontoid process of axis

Nasal part of pharynx

Spinous process of axis

Soft palate

Anterior arch of atlas

Oral cavity

Mental protuberance

Mandibular angle (ipsilateral)

Hyoid bone

Mandibular angle (contralateral)

Condylar process of mandible (ipsilateral)

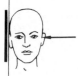

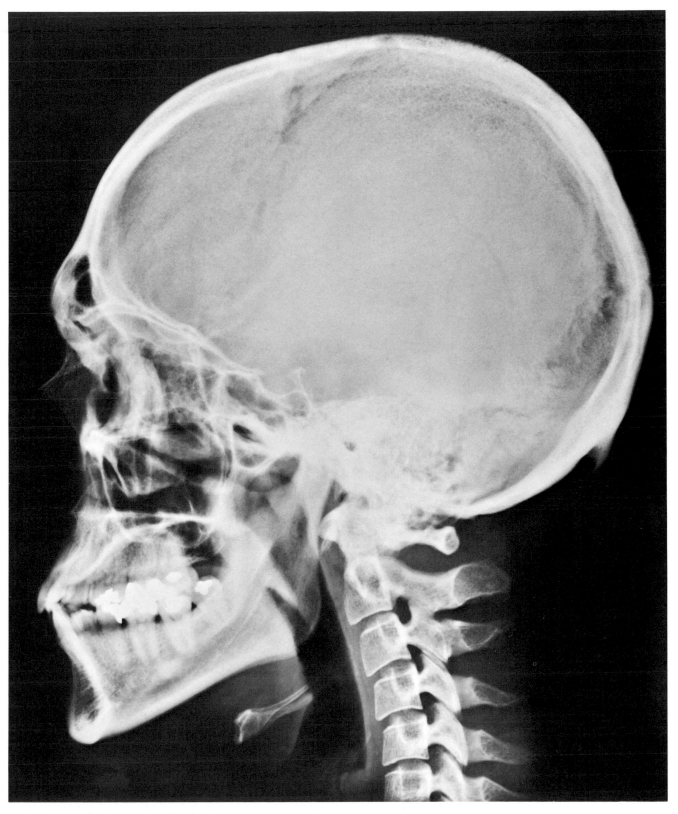

Fig. 3. Skull (lateral projection)

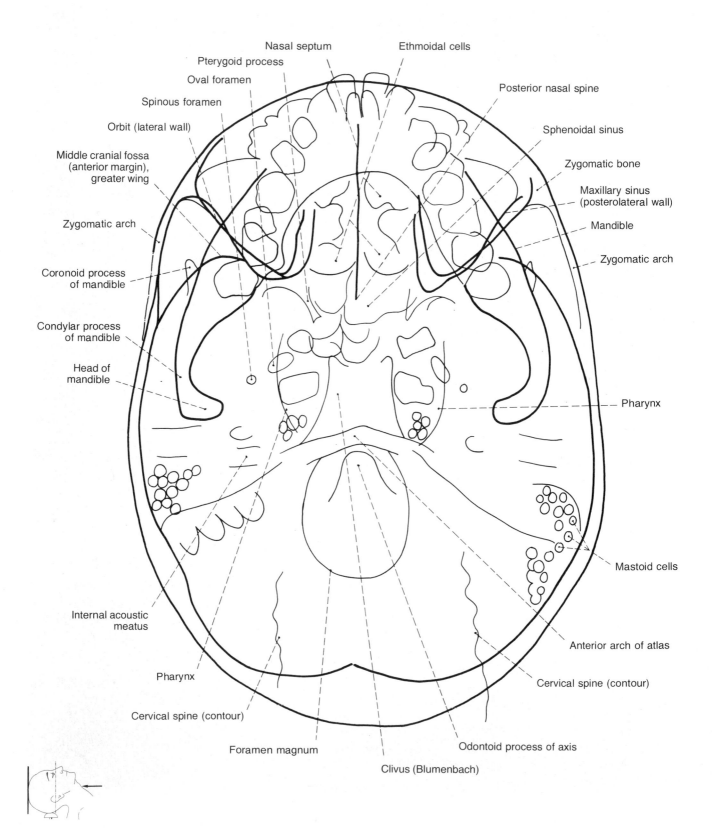

Nasal septum

Ethmoidal cells

Pterygoid process

Oval foramen

Posterior nasal spine

Spinous foramen

Orbit (lateral wall)

Sphenoidal sinus

Middle cranial fossa
(anterior margin),
greater wing

Zygomatic bone

Maxillary sinus
(posterolateral wall)

Zygomatic arch

Mandible

Coronoid process
of mandible

Zygomatic arch

Condylar process
of mandible

Head of
mandible

Pharynx

Mastoid cells

Internal acoustic
meatus

Anterior arch of atlas

Pharynx

Cervical spine (contour)

Cervical spine (contour)

Foramen magnum

Odontoid process of axis

Clivus (Blumenbach)

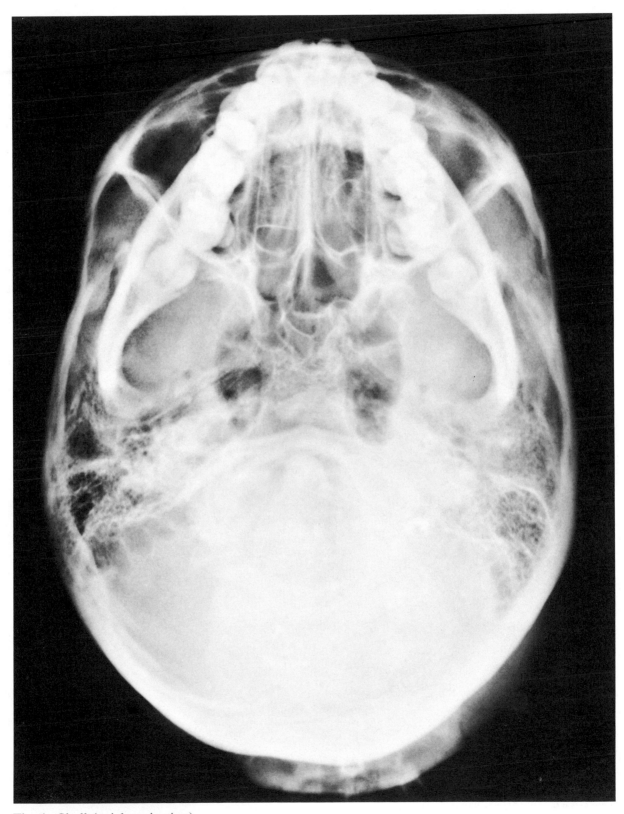

Fig. 4. Skull (axial projection)

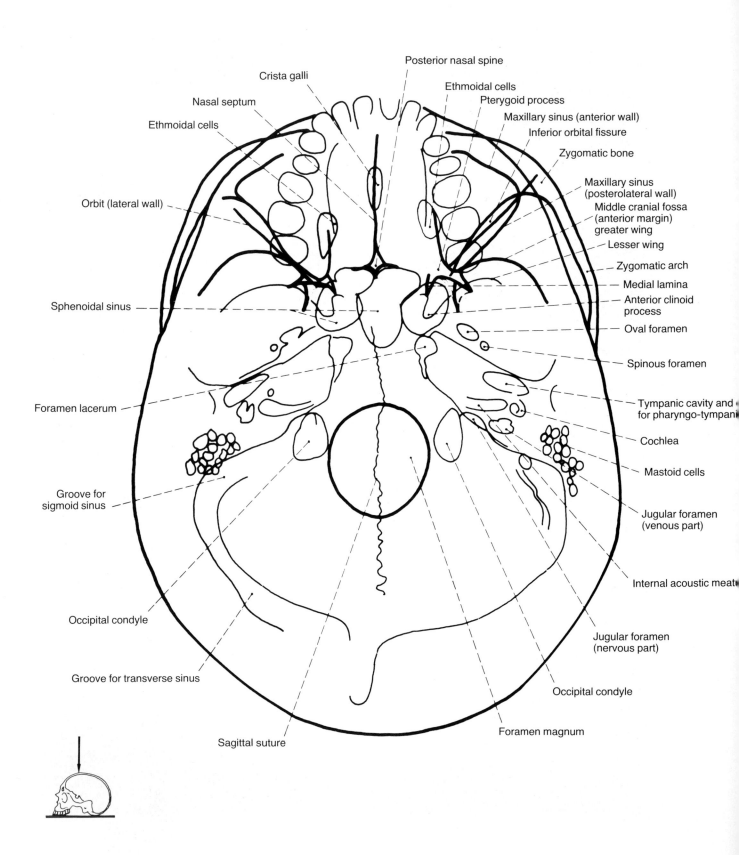

Posterior nasal spine

Crista galli

Nasal septum

Ethmoidal cells

Ethmoidal cells

Pterygoid process

Maxillary sinus (anterior wall)

Inferior orbital fissure

Zygomatic bone

Orbit (lateral wall)

Maxillary sinus (posterolateral wall)

Middle cranial fossa (anterior margin) greater wing

Lesser wing

Zygomatic arch

Medial lamina

Anterior clinoid process

Sphenoidal sinus

Oval foramen

Spinous foramen

Tympanic cavity and for pharyngo-tympani

Cochlea

Foramen lacerum

Mastoid cells

Jugular foramen (venous part)

Groove for sigmoid sinus

Internal acoustic meat

Occipital condyle

Jugular foramen (nervous part)

Groove for transverse sinus

Occipital condyle

Sagittal suture

Foramen magnum

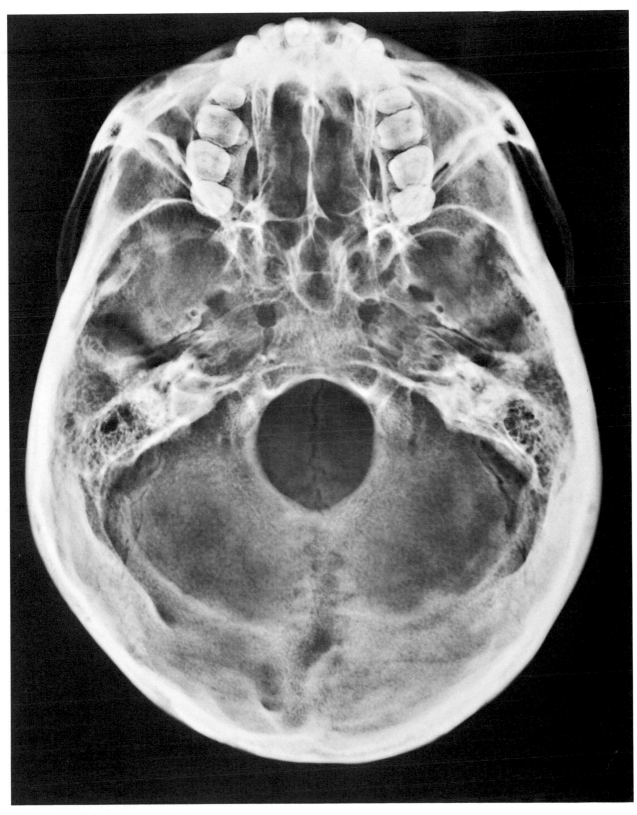

Fig. 5. Skull (axial projection)

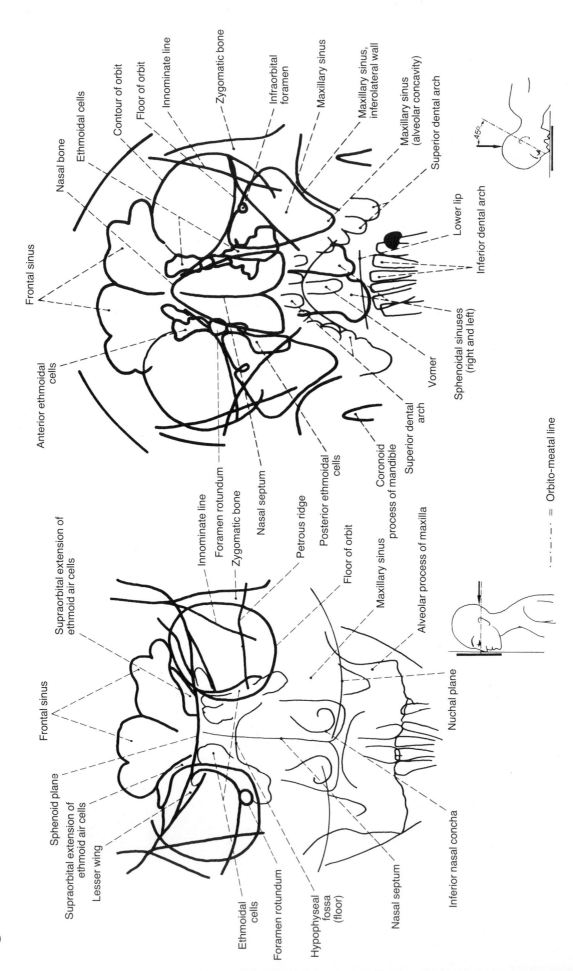

Frontal sinus

Anterior ethmoidal cells

Nasal bone

Ethmoidal cells

Contour of orbit

Floor of orbit

Innominate line

Zygomatic bone

Infraorbital foramen

Maxillary sinus

Maxillary sinus, inferolateral wall

Maxillary sinus (alveolar concavity)

Superior dental arch

Lower lip

Inferior dental arch

Vomer

Sphenoidal sinuses (right and left)

Superior dental arch

Coronoid process of mandible

Posterior ethmoidal cells

Floor of orbit

Maxillary sinus

Alveolar process of maxilla

Nasal septum

Petrous ridge

Zygomatic bone

Foramen rotundum

Innominate line

Supraorbital extension of ethmoid air cells

Frontal sinus

Sphenoid plane

Supraorbital extension of ethmoid air cells

Lesser wing

Ethmoidal cells

Foramen rotundum

Hypophyseal fossa (floor)

Nasal septum

Inferior nasal concha

Nuchal plane

Orbito-meatal line

45°

- · - · - =  Orbito-meatal line

10

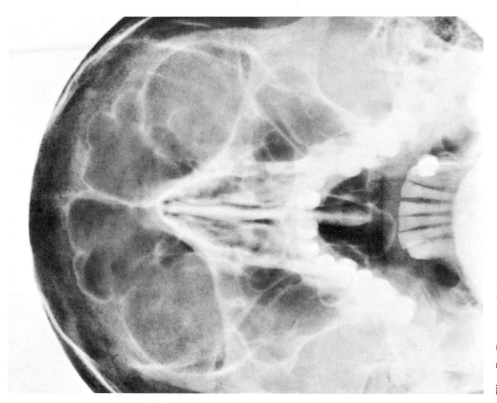

Fig. 7. Paranasal sinuses (Water's projection)

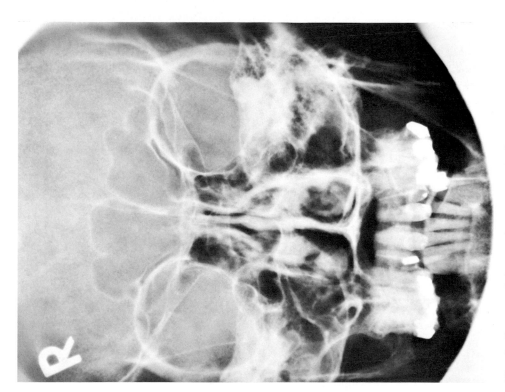

Fig. 6. Paranasal sinuses (p.a. projection)

# Paranasal Sinuses, Orbitae

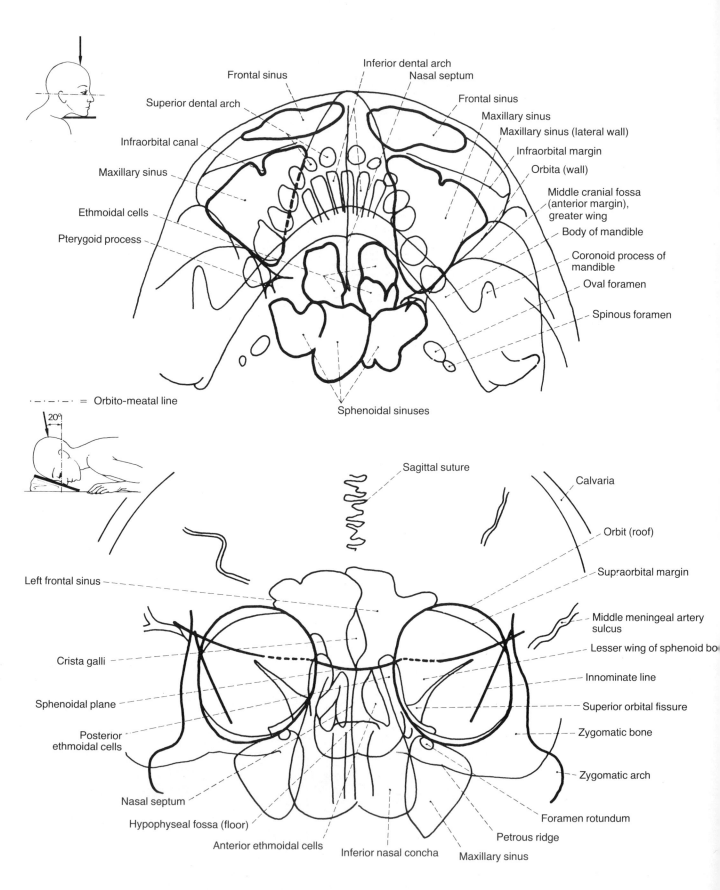

Frontal sinus

Inferior dental arch

Nasal septum

Superior dental arch

Frontal sinus

Maxillary sinus

Maxillary sinus (lateral wall)

Infraorbital canal

Infraorbital margin

Maxillary sinus

Orbita (wall)

Middle cranial fossa (anterior margin), greater wing

Ethmoidal cells

Body of mandible

Pterygoid process

Coronoid process of mandible

Oval foramen

Spinous foramen

Sphenoidal sinuses

- · - · - · - · - = Orbito-meatal line

20°

Sagittal suture

Calvaria

Orbit (roof)

Left frontal sinus

Supraorbital margin

Middle meningeal artery sulcus

Crista galli

Lesser wing of sphenoid bo

Sphenoidal plane

Innominate line

Posterior ethmoidal cells

Superior orbital fissure

Zygomatic bone

Nasal septum

Zygomatic arch

Hypophyseal fossa (floor)

Foramen rotundum

Anterior ethmoidal cells

Petrous ridge

Inferior nasal concha

Maxillary sinus

12

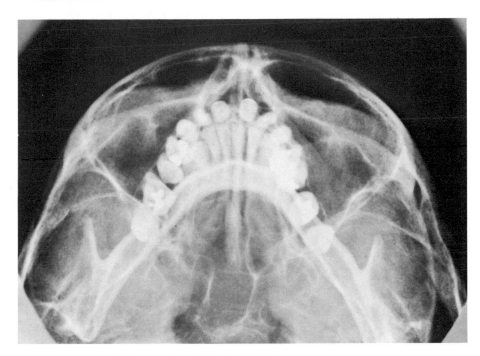

Fig. 8. Paranasal sinuses (axial projection)

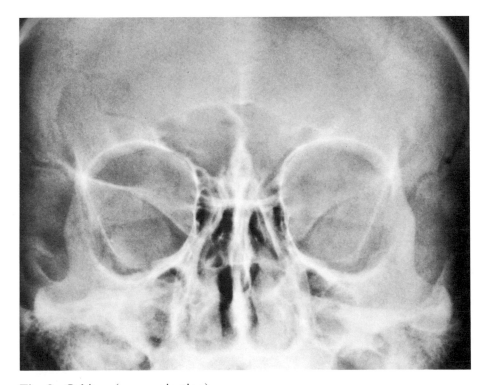

Fig. 9. Orbitae (p.a. projection)

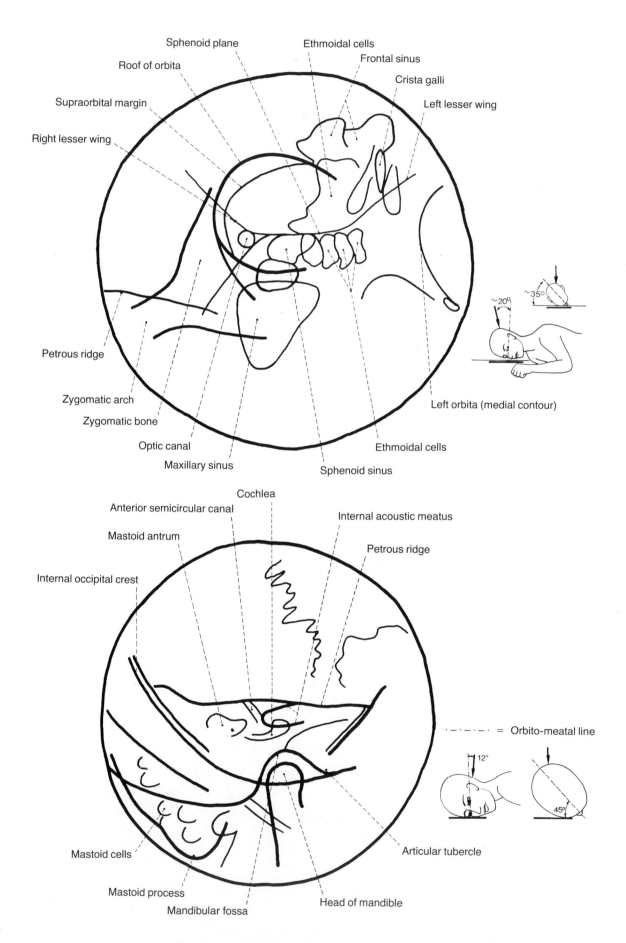

Sphenoid plane
Roof of orbita
Supraorbital margin
Right lesser wing
Ethmoidal cells
Frontal sinus
Crista galli
Left lesser wing

~20°   ~35°

Petrous ridge
Zygomatic arch
Zygomatic bone
Optic canal
Maxillary sinus
Sphenoid sinus
Ethmoidal cells
Left orbita (medial contour)

Cochlea
Anterior semicircular canal
Mastoid antrum
Internal occipital crest
Internal acoustic meatus
Petrous ridge

—·—·— = Orbito-meatal line

12°
45°

Mastoid cells
Mastoid process
Mandibular fossa
Head of mandible
Articular tubercle

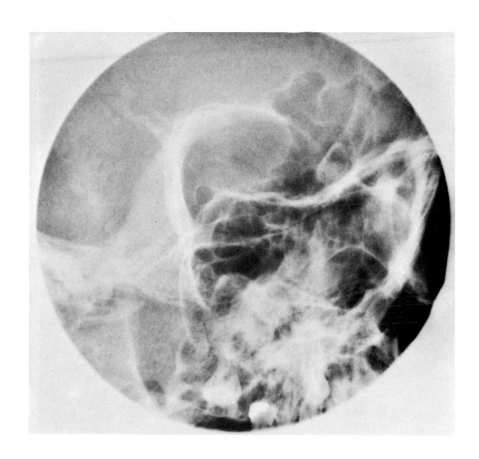

Fig. 10. Radiograph
of right canalis opticus (Rhese)

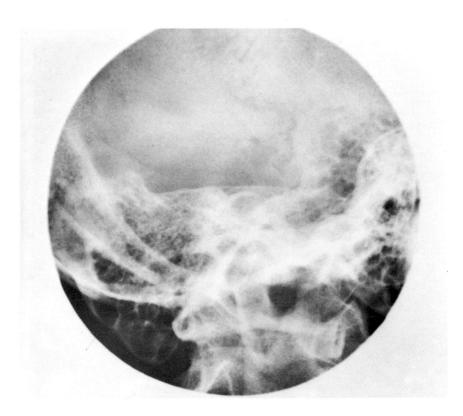

Fig. 11. Semisagittal radiograph
of right temporal bone (Stenvers)

# Temporal Bone

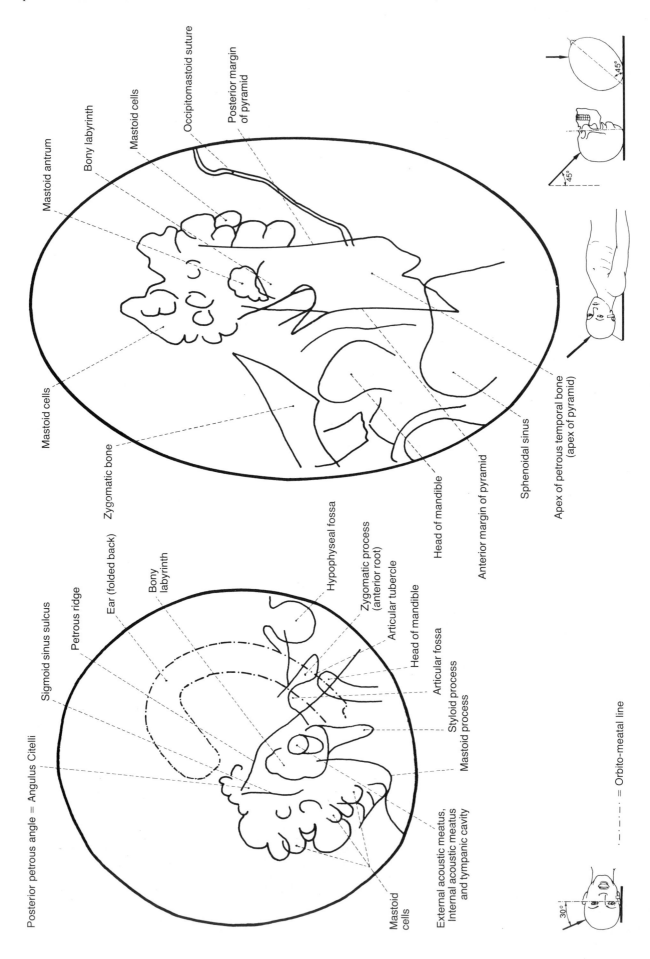

Mastoid antrum

Bony labyrinth

Mastoid cells

Occipitomastoid suture

Posterior margin of pyramid

Mastoid cells

Zygomatic bone

Apex of petrous temporal bone (apex of pyramid)

Sphenoidal sinus

Anterior margin of pyramid

Head of mandible

Hypophyseal fossa

Zygomatic process (anterior root)

Articular tubercle

Head of mandible

Articular fossa

Styloid process

Mastoid process

Sigmoid sinus sulcus

Petrous ridge

Ear (folded back)

Bony labyrinth

Posterior petrous angle = Angulus Citelli

Mastoid cells

External acoustic meatus, Internal acoustic meatus and tympanic cavity

– · – · – = Orbito-meatal line

45°

45°

30°

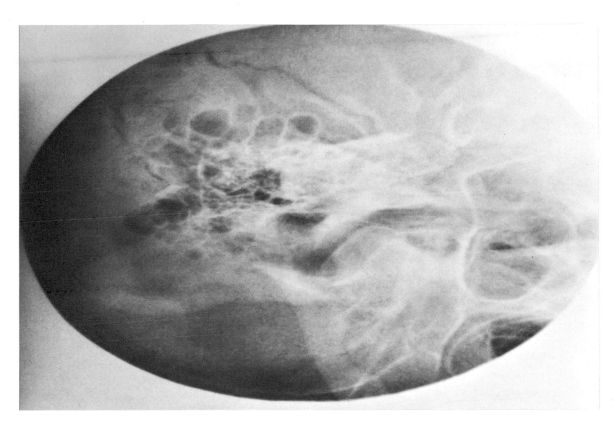

Fig. 13. Radiograph of left temporal bone
(semiaxial projection, Mayer)

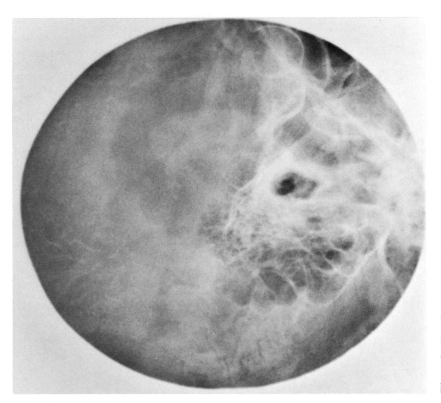

Fig. 12. Radiograph of right temporal bone
(semilateral projection, Schüller)

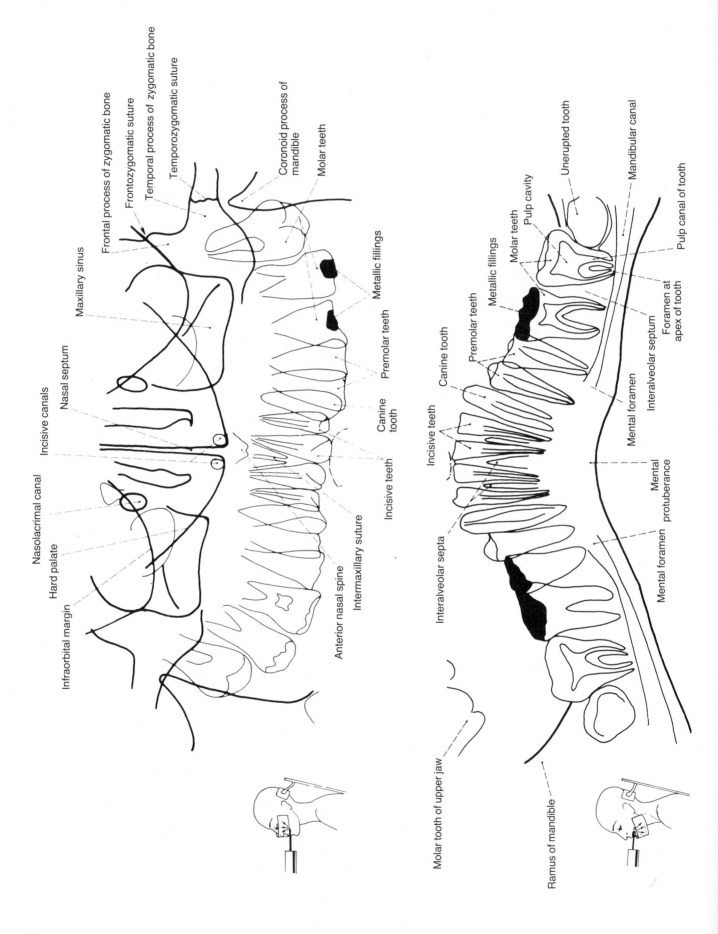

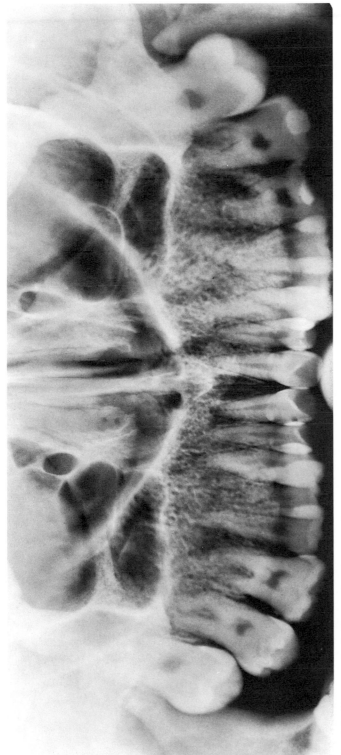

Fig. 14. Panoramic radiograph of upper jaw

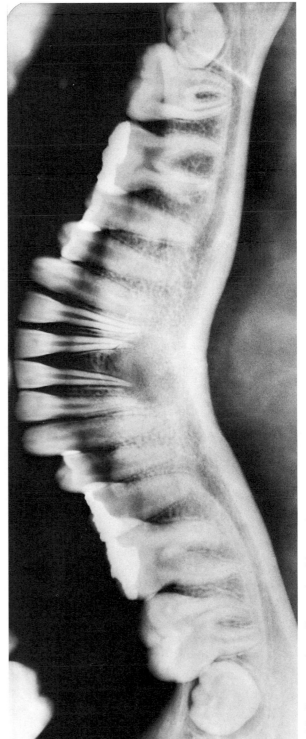

Fig. 15. Panoramic radiograph of lower jaw

# Carotid Angiography

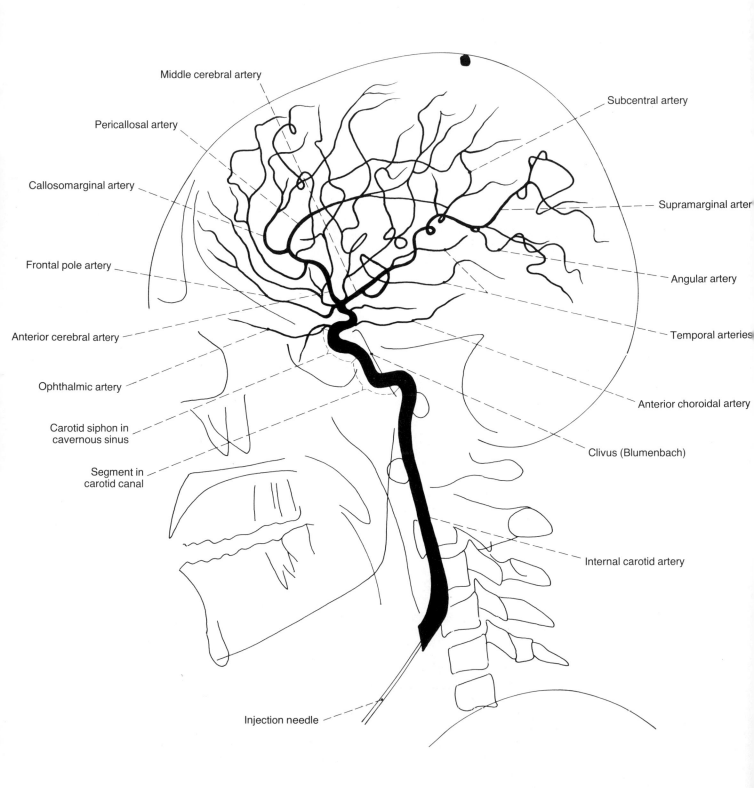

Middle cerebral artery

Pericallosal artery

Callosomarginal artery

Frontal pole artery

Anterior cerebral artery

Ophthalmic artery

Carotid siphon in cavernous sinus

Segment in carotid canal

Subcentral artery

Supramarginal artery

Angular artery

Temporal arteries

Anterior choroidal artery

Clivus (Blumenbach)

Internal carotid artery

Injection needle

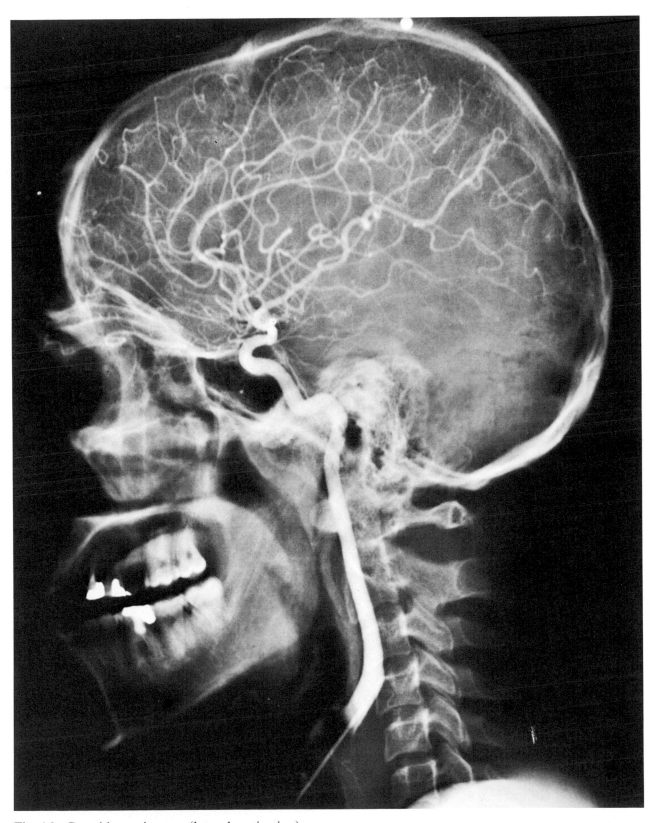

Fig. 16. Carotid arteriogram (lateral projection)

# Carotid Angiography

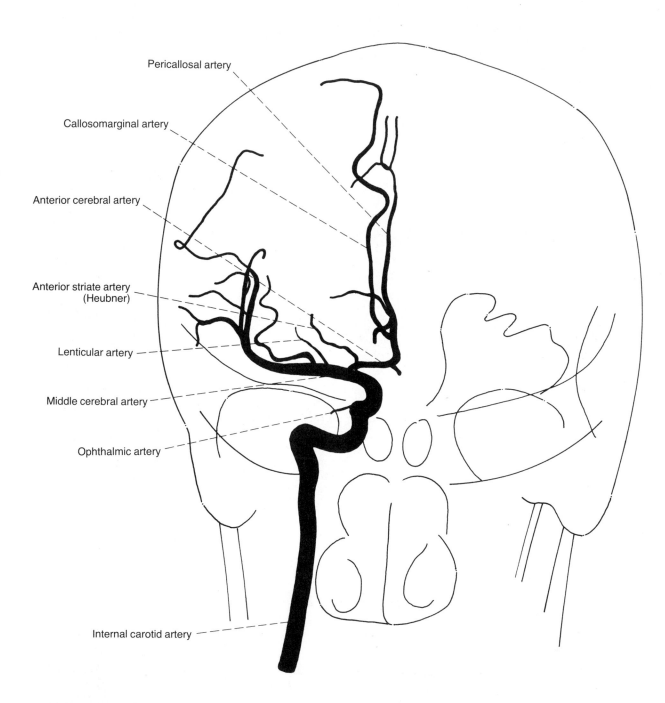

Pericallosal artery

Callosomarginal artery

Anterior cerebral artery

Anterior striate artery
(Heubner)

Lenticular artery

Middle cerebral artery

Ophthalmic artery

Internal carotid artery

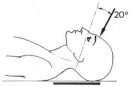

20°

$- \cdot - \cdot - \cdot -$ = Orbito-meatal line

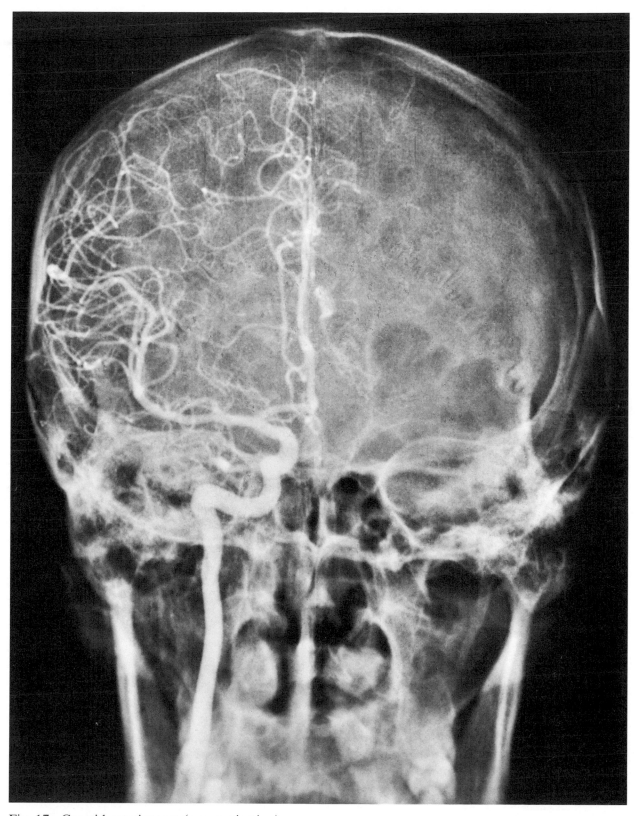

Fig. 17. Carotid arteriogram (a.p. projection)

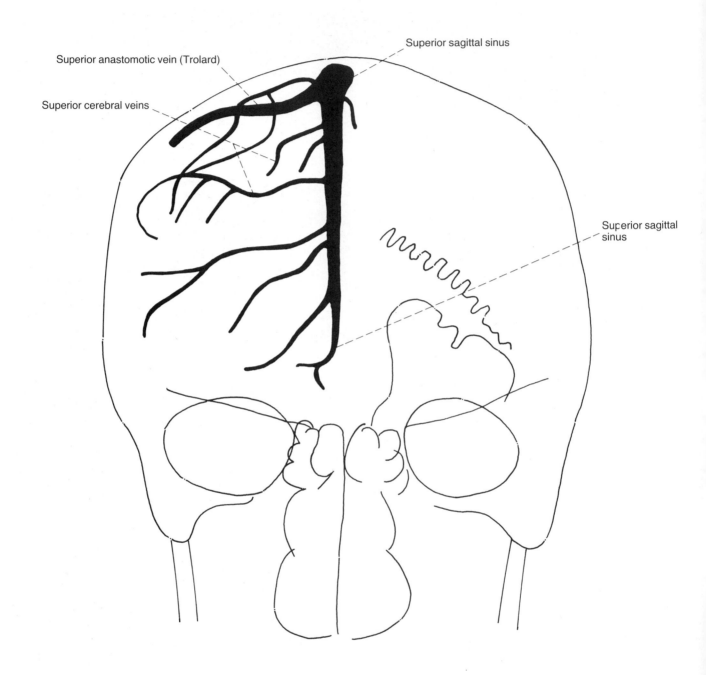

Superior sagittal sinus

Superior anastomotic vein (Trolard)

Superior cerebral veins

Superior sagittal sinus

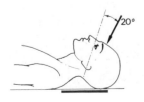

20°

·—·—·— = Orbito-meatal line

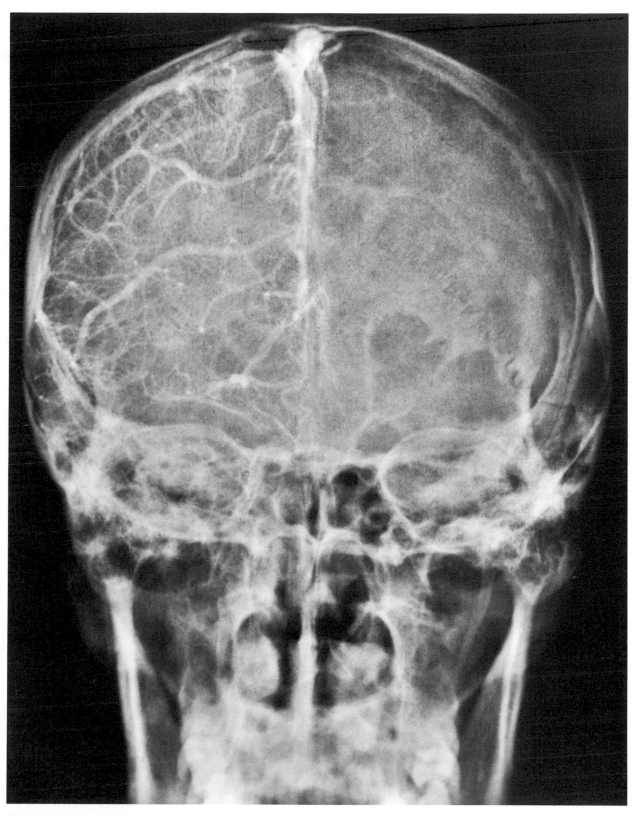

Fig. 18.  Carotid arteriogram, venous phase (a.p. projection)

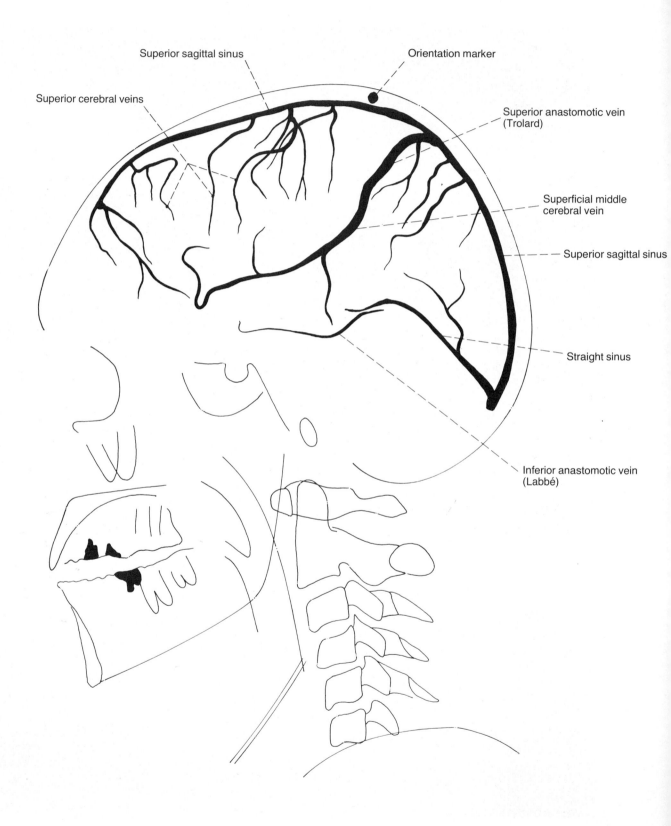

Superior sagittal sinus

Orientation marker

Superior cerebral veins

Superior anastomotic vein
(Trolard)

Superficial middle
cerebral vein

Superior sagittal sinus

Straight sinus

Inferior anastomotic vein
(Labbé)

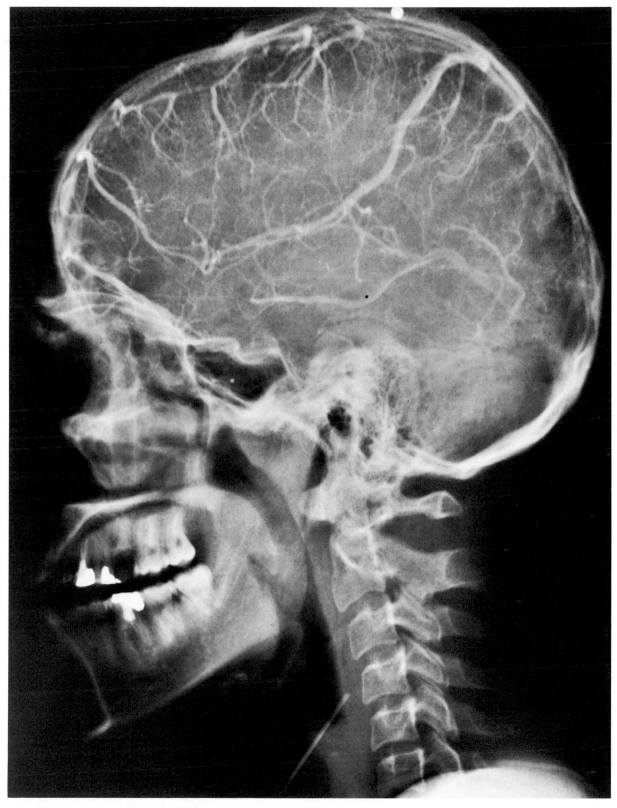

Fig. 19. Carotid arteriogram, venous phase (lateral projection)

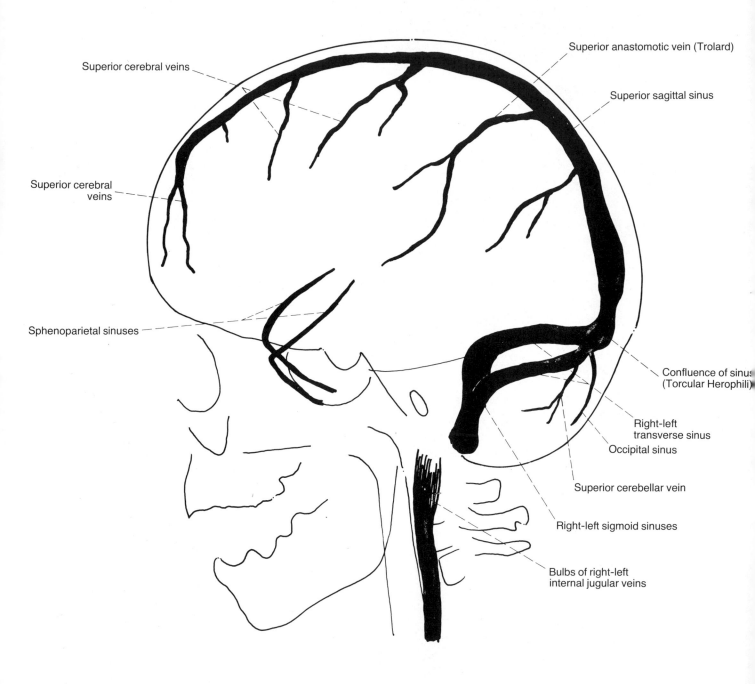

Superior cerebral veins

Superior anastomotic vein (Trolard)

Superior sagittal sinus

Superior cerebral veins

Sphenoparietal sinuses

Confluence of sinus (Torcular Herophili)

Right-left transverse sinus

Occipital sinus

Superior cerebellar vein

Right-left sigmoid sinuses

Bulbs of right-left internal jugular veins

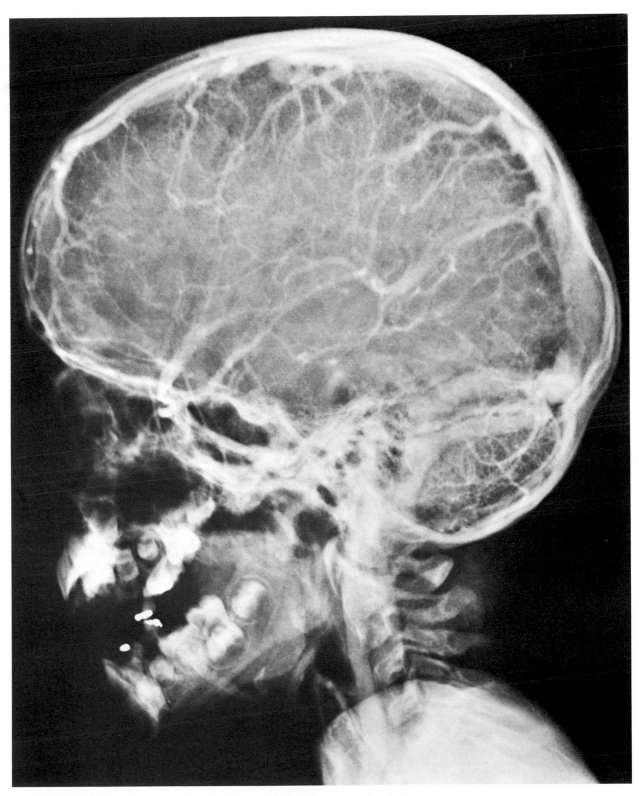

Fig. 20. Carotid arteriogram, late venous phase (lateral projection)

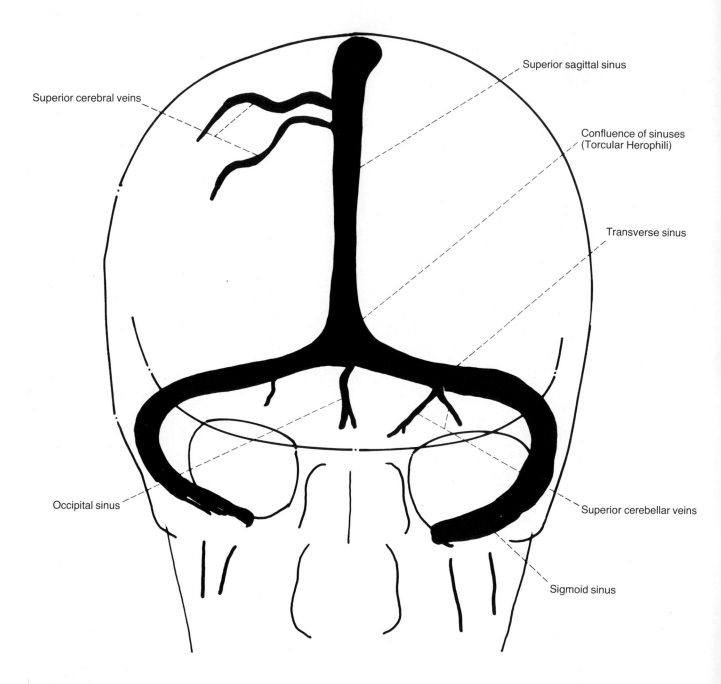

Superior cerebral veins

Superior sagittal sinus

Confluence of sinuses
(Torcular Herophili)

Transverse sinus

Occipital sinus

Superior cerebellar veins

Sigmoid sinus

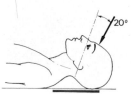

20°

— · — · — = Orbito-meatal line

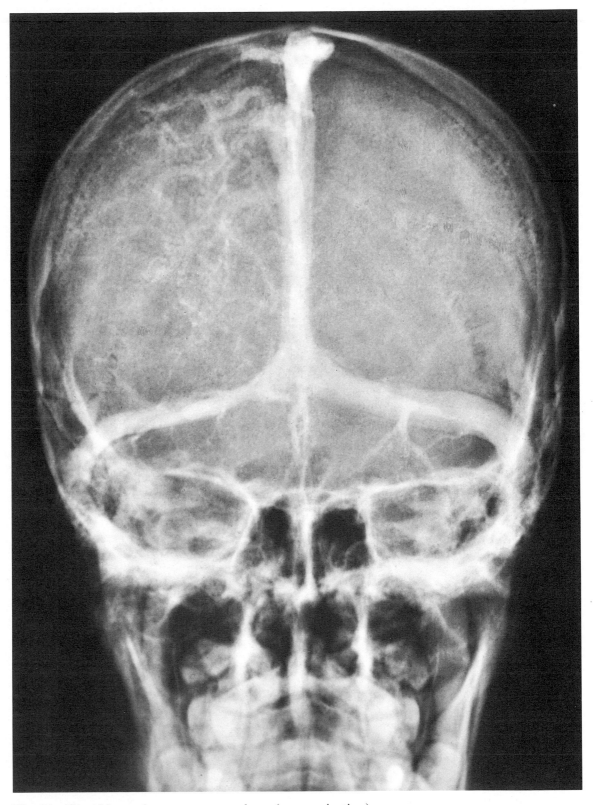

Fig. 21. Carotid arteriogram, venous phase (a.p. projection)

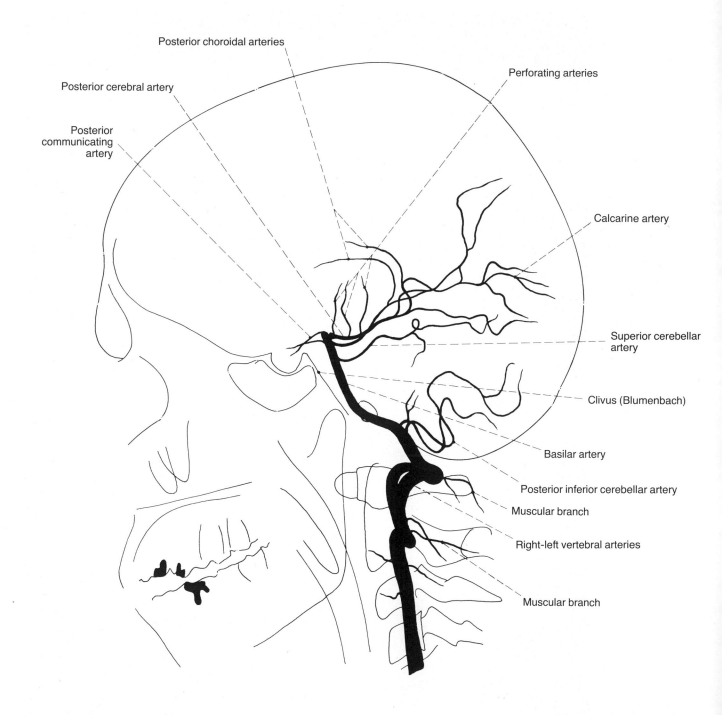

Posterior choroidal arteries

Perforating arteries

Posterior cerebral artery

Posterior communicating artery

Calcarine artery

Superior cerebellar artery

Clivus (Blumenbach)

Basilar artery

Posterior inferior cerebellar artery

Muscular branch

Right-left vertebral arteries

Muscular branch

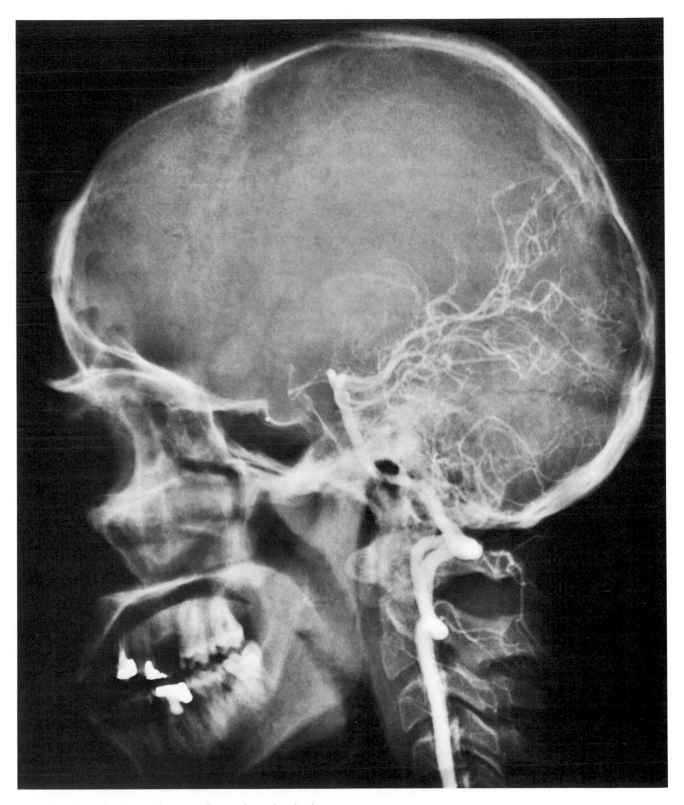

Fig. 22. Vertebral arteriogram (lateral projection)

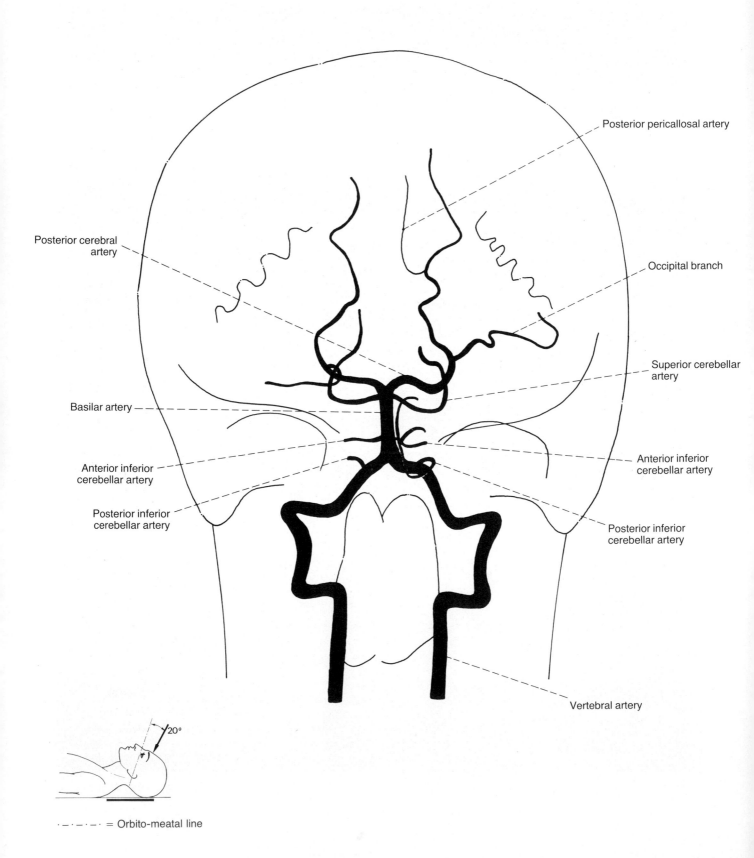

Posterior pericallosal artery

Posterior cerebral artery

Occipital branch

Superior cerebellar artery

Basilar artery

Anterior inferior cerebellar artery

Anterior inferior cerebellar artery

Posterior inferior cerebellar artery

Posterior inferior cerebellar artery

Vertebral artery

20°

- · - · - · - = Orbito-meatal line

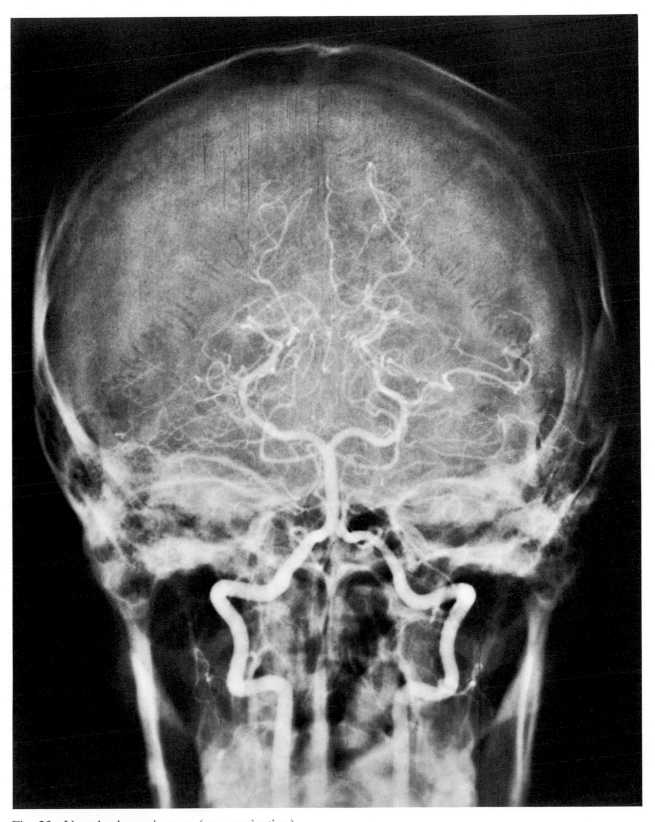

Fig. 23. Vertebral arteriogram (a.p. projection)

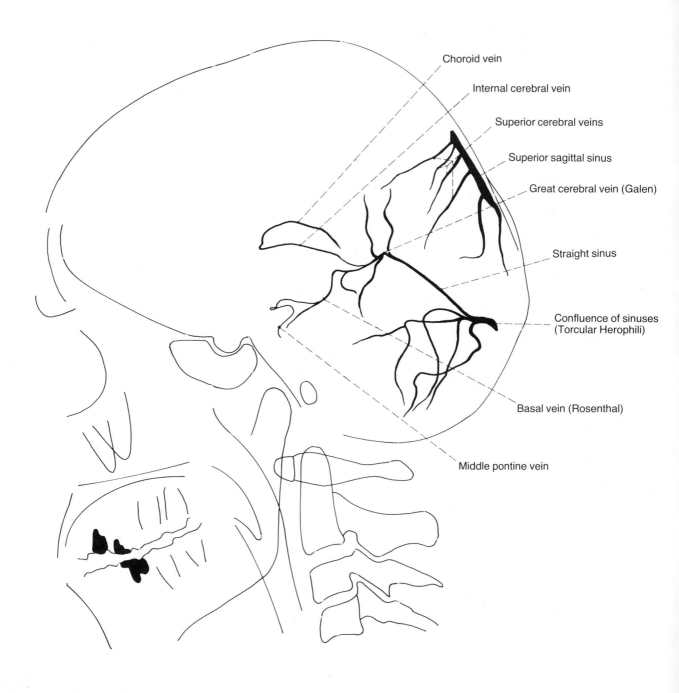

Choroid vein

Internal cerebral vein

Superior cerebral veins

Superior sagittal sinus

Great cerebral vein (Galen)

Straight sinus

Confluence of sinuses
(Torcular Herophili)

Basal vein (Rosenthal)

Middle pontine vein

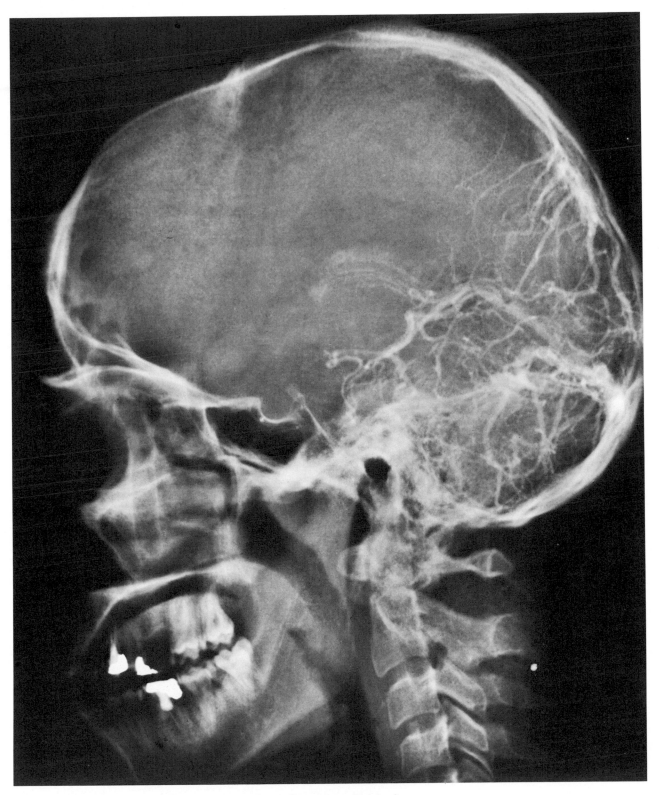

Fig. 24. Vertebral arteriogram, venous phase (lateral projection)

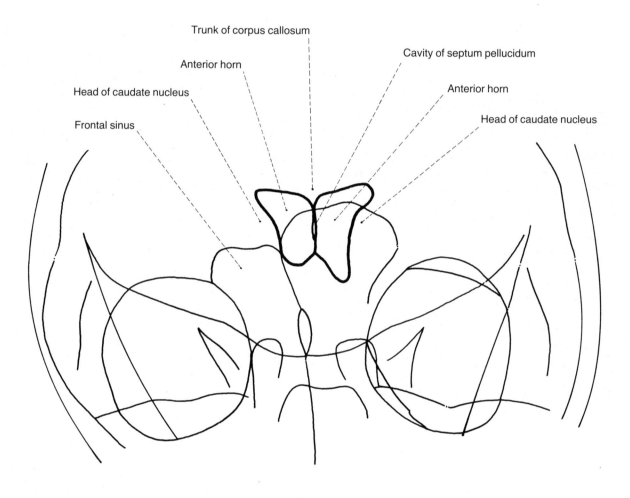

Trunk of corpus callosum

Anterior horn

Cavity of septum pellucidum

Head of caudate nucleus

Anterior horn

Frontal sinus

Head of caudate nucleus

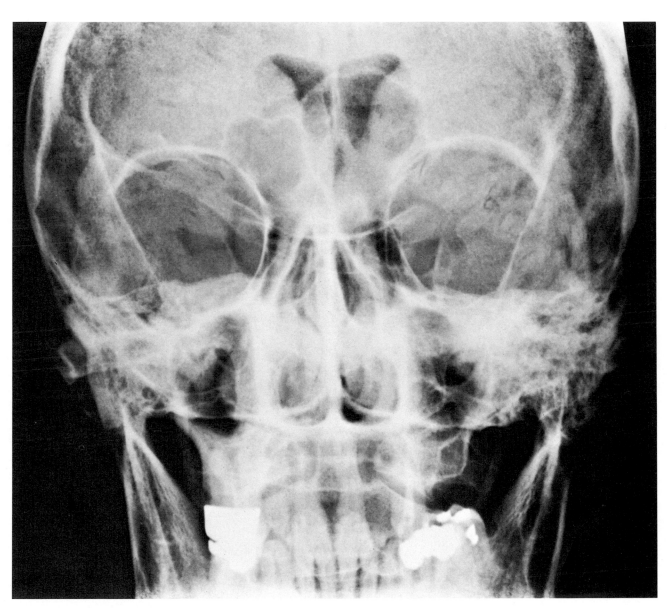

Fig. 25.  Ventriculogram (a.p. projection)

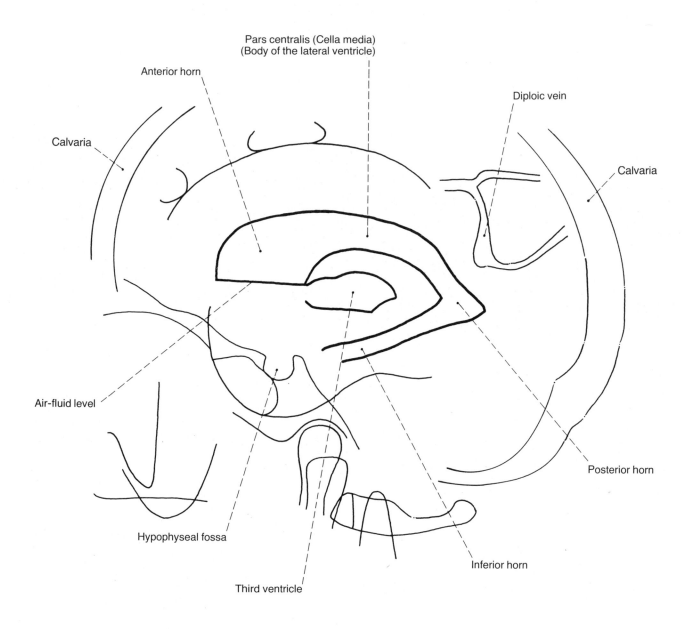

Pars centralis (Cella media)
(Body of the lateral ventricle)

Anterior horn

Diploic vein

Calvaria

Calvaria

Air-fluid level

Hypophyseal fossa

Posterior horn

Third ventricle

Inferior horn

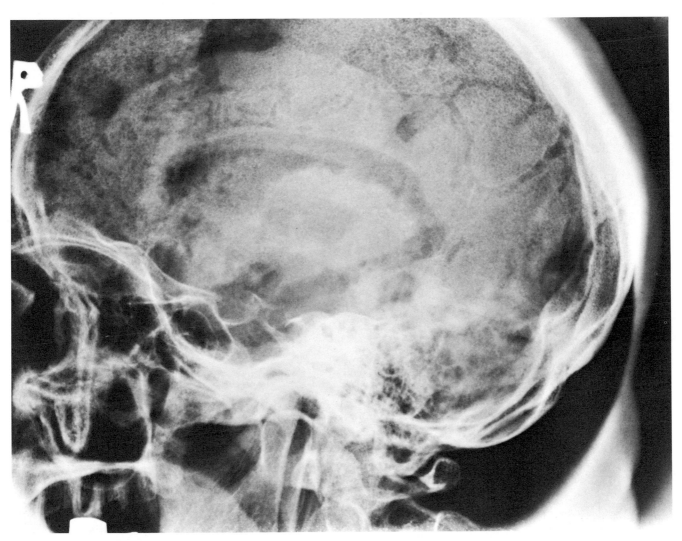

Fig. 26. Ventriculogram (lateral projection)

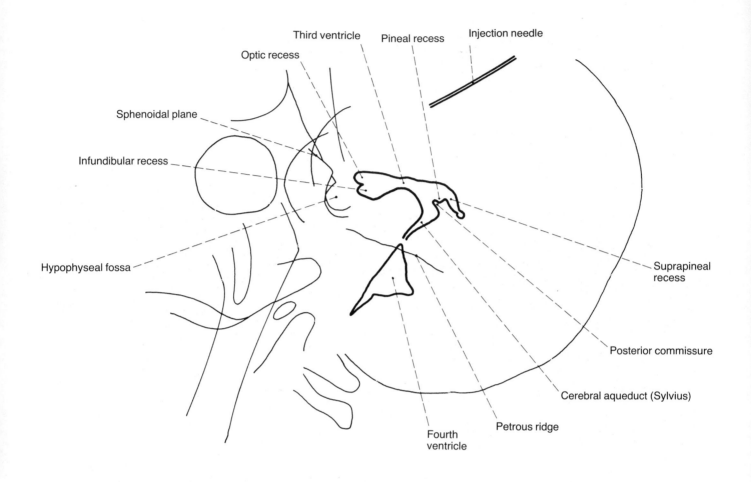

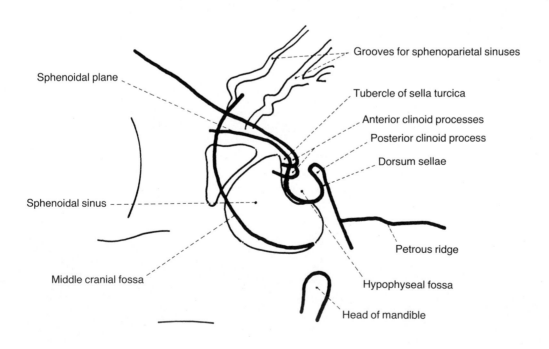

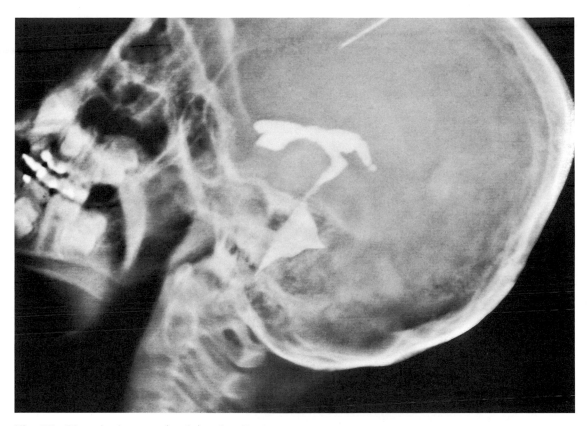

Fig. 27. Ventriculogram (path.) using Pantopaque

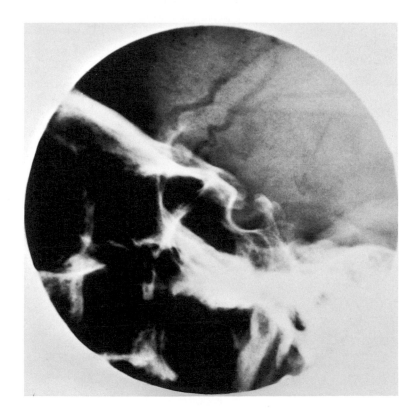

Fig. 28. Radiograph, coned-down view
of sella turcica

# Spinal Column

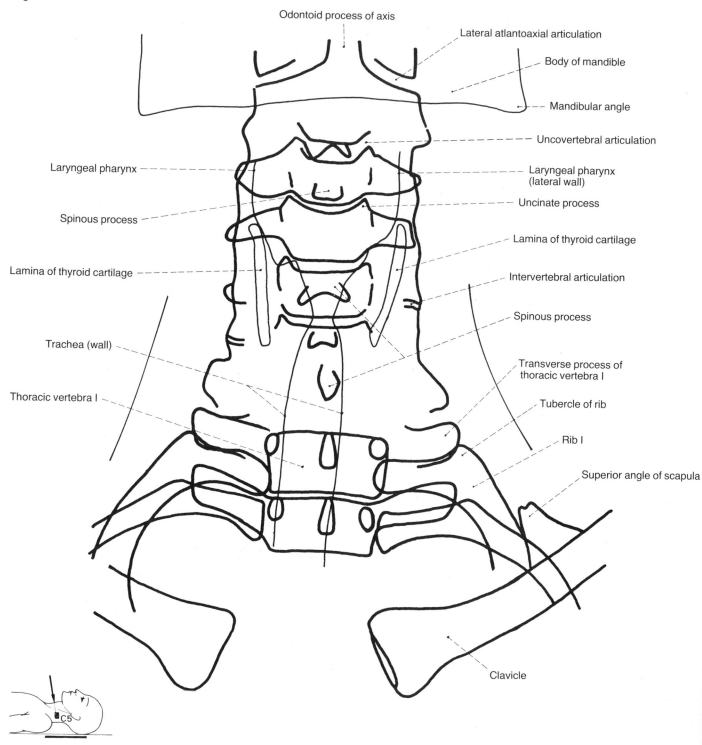

Odontoid process of axis

Lateral atlantoaxial articulation

Body of mandible

Mandibular angle

Uncovertebral articulation

Laryngeal pharynx

Laryngeal pharynx
(lateral wall)

Uncinate process

Spinous process

Lamina of thyroid cartilage

Lamina of thyroid cartilage

Intervertebral articulation

Spinous process

Trachea (wall)

Transverse process of
thoracic vertebra I

Thoracic vertebra I

Tubercle of rib

Rib I

Superior angle of scapula

Clavicle

C5

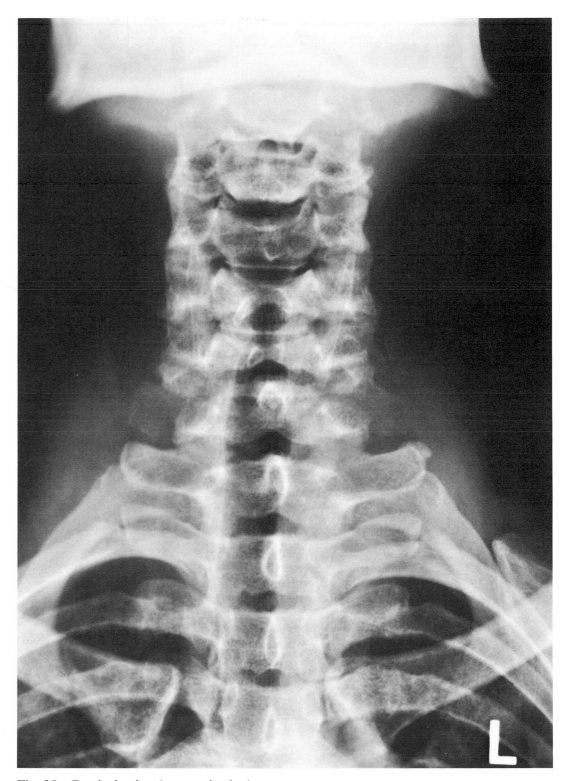

Fig. 29.  Cervical spine (a.p. projection)

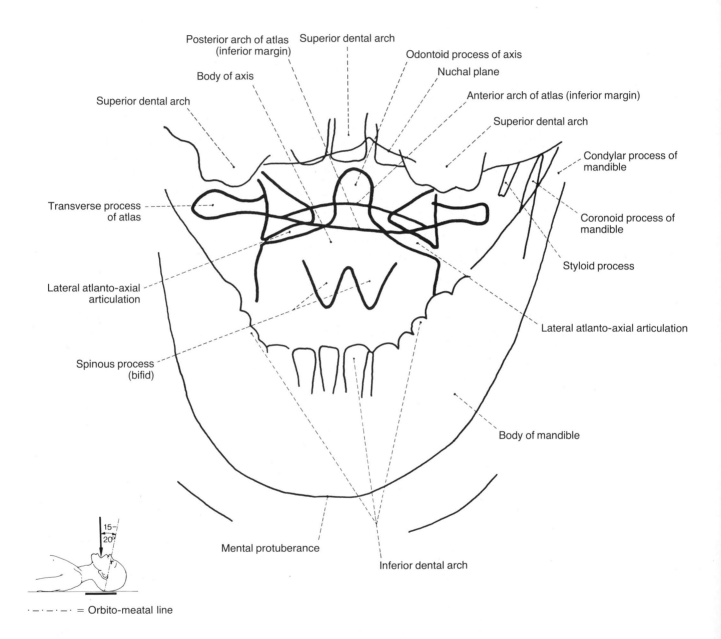

Posterior arch of atlas
(inferior margin)

Superior dental arch

Odontoid process of axis

Body of axis

Nuchal plane

Anterior arch of atlas (inferior margin)

Superior dental arch

Superior dental arch

Condylar process of
mandible

Transverse process
of atlas

Coronoid process of
mandible

Styloid process

Lateral atlanto-axial
articulation

Lateral atlanto-axial articulation

Body of mandible

Spinous process
(bifid)

Mental protuberance

Inferior dental arch

15–
20°

· – · – · – · = Orbito-meatal line

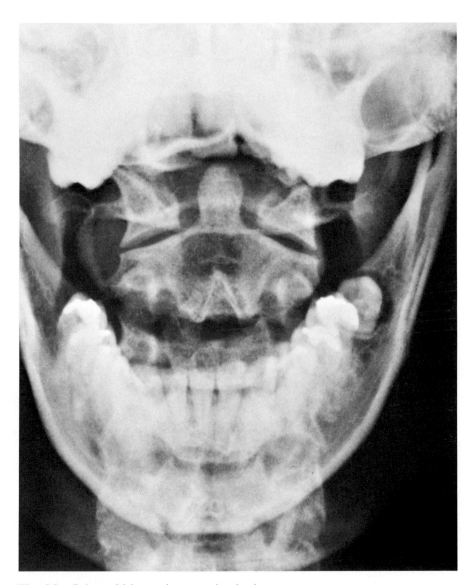

Fig. 30. Odontoid bone (a.p. projection)

# Cervical Spine

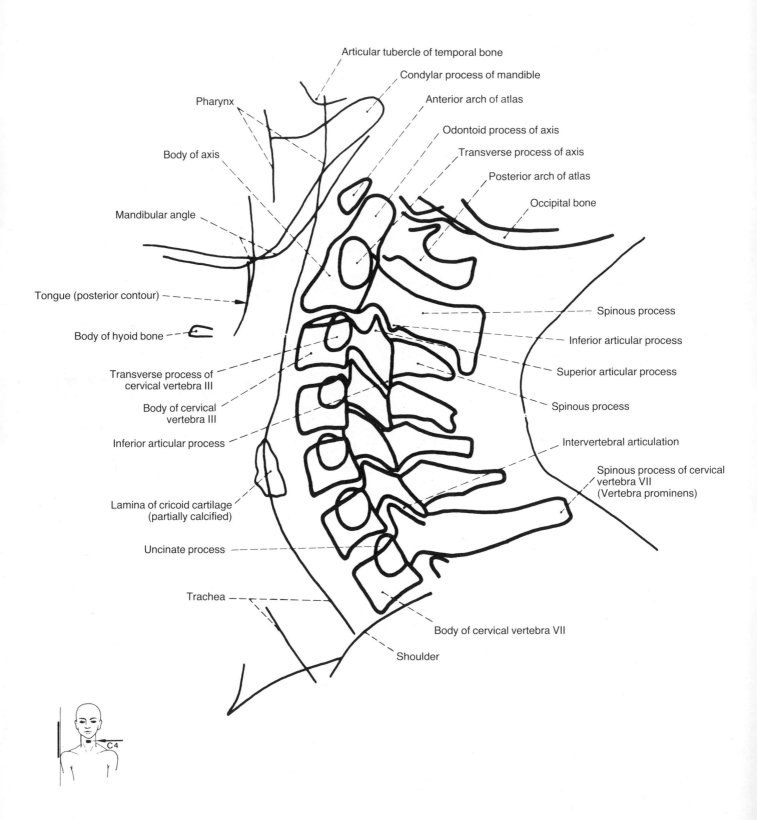

Articular tubercle of temporal bone

Condylar process of mandible

Pharynx

Anterior arch of atlas

Odontoid process of axis

Body of axis

Transverse process of axis

Posterior arch of atlas

Occipital bone

Mandibular angle

Tongue (posterior contour)

Spinous process

Body of hyoid bone

Inferior articular process

Superior articular process

Transverse process of cervical vertebra III

Body of cervical vertebra III

Spinous process

Inferior articular process

Intervertebral articulation

Spinous process of cervical vertebra VII (Vertebra prominens)

Lamina of cricoid cartilage (partially calcified)

Uncinate process

Trachea

Body of cervical vertebra VII

Shoulder

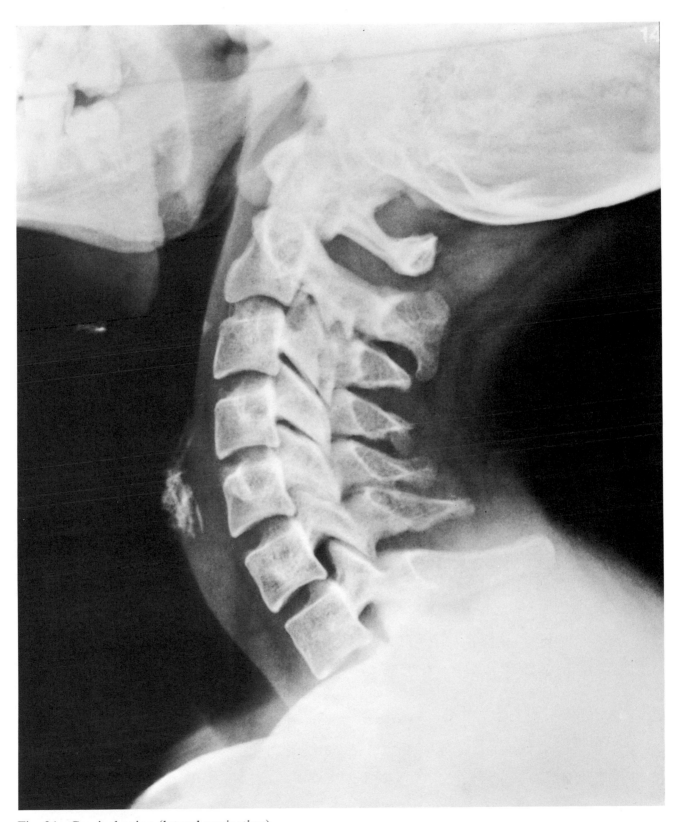

Fig. 31. Cervical spine (lateral projection)

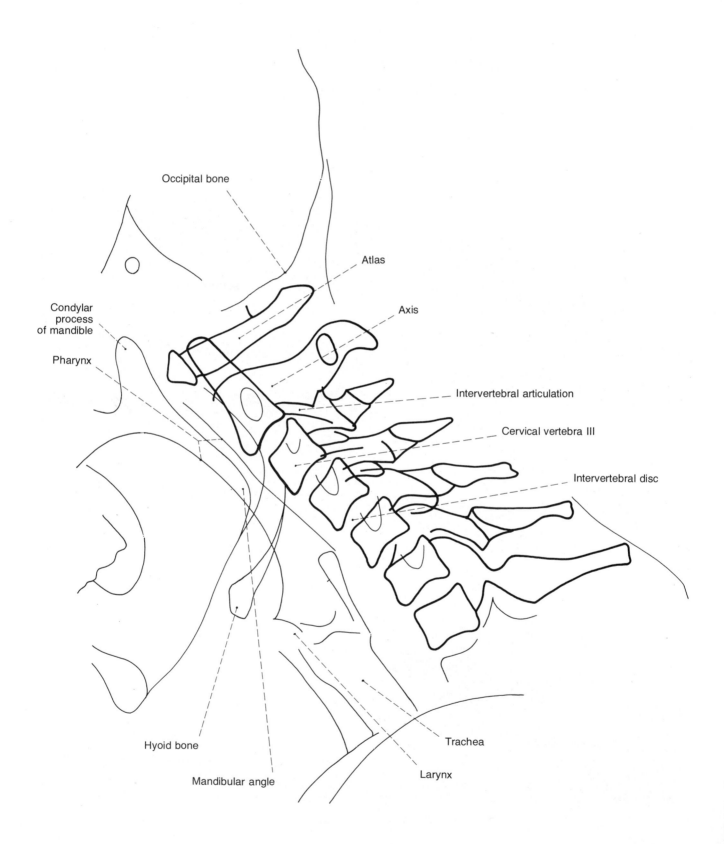

Occipital bone

Atlas

Axis

Condylar
process
of mandible

Pharynx

Intervertebral articulation

Cervical vertebra III

Intervertebral disc

Hyoid bone

Mandibular angle

Trachea

Larynx

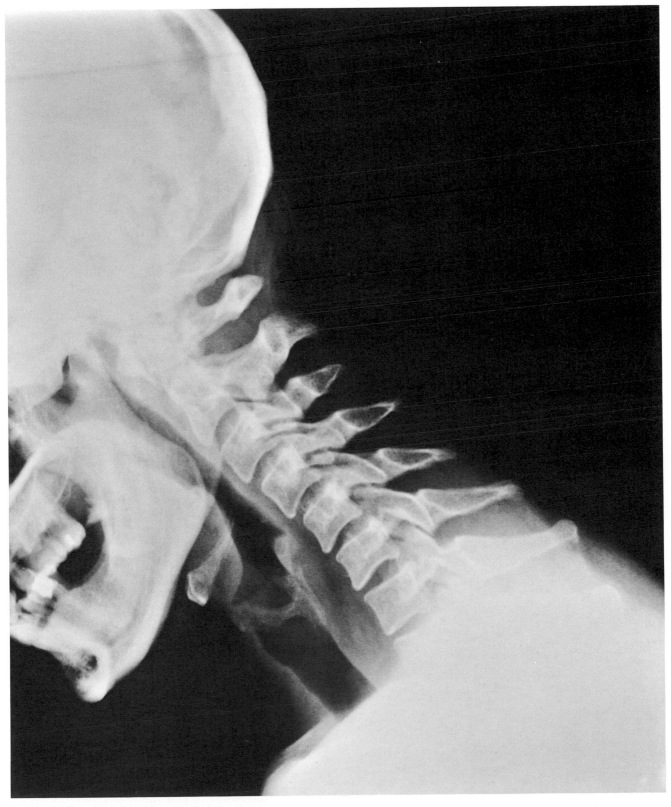

Fig. 32. Cervical spine, functional exposure with extreme anteflexion

# Cervical Spine

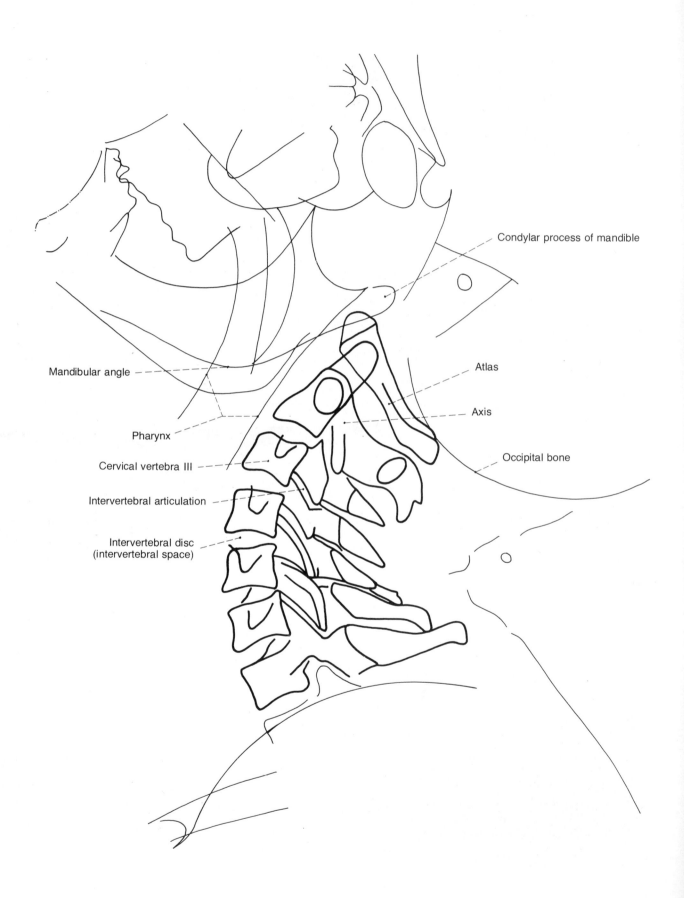

Condylar process of mandible

Mandibular angle

Atlas

Axis

Pharynx

Occipital bone

Cervical vertebra III

Intervertebral articulation

Intervertebral disc
(intervertebral space)

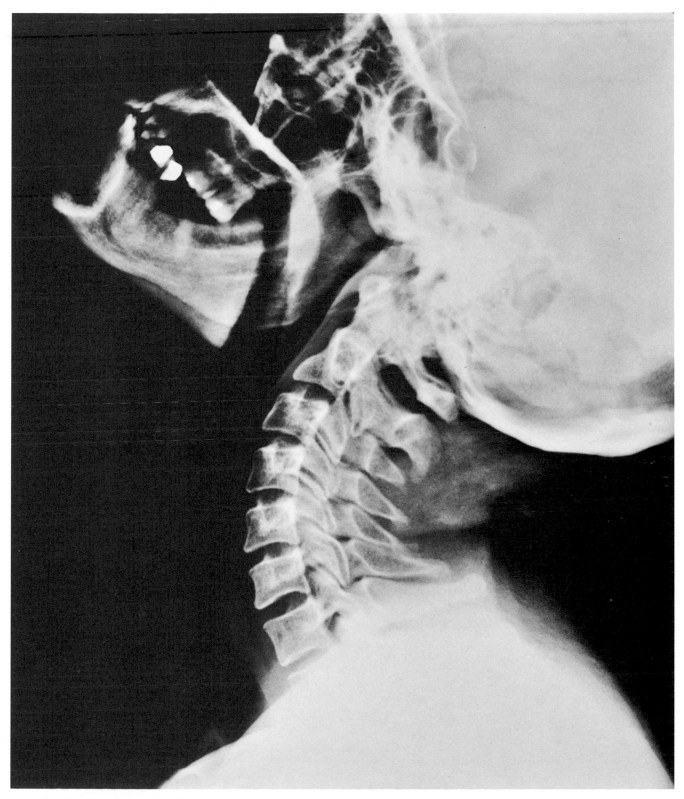

Fig. 33. Cervical spine, functional exposure with extreme retroflexion

# Cervical Spine

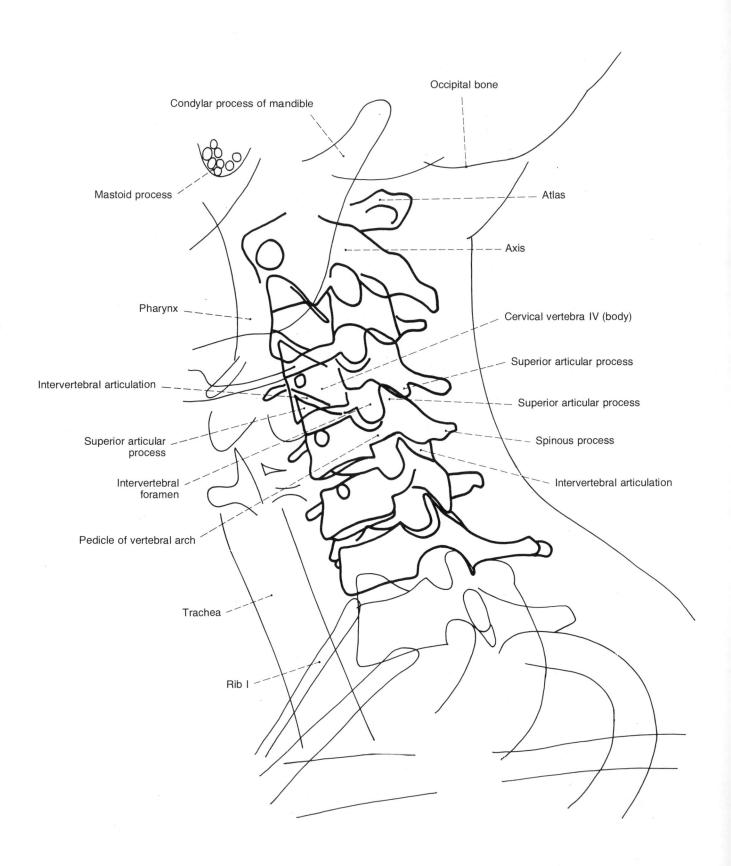

Condylar process of mandible

Occipital bone

Mastoid process

Atlas

Axis

Pharynx

Cervical vertebra IV (body)

Superior articular process

Intervertebral articulation

Superior articular process

Superior articular process

Spinous process

Intervertebral foramen

Intervertebral articulation

Pedicle of vertebral arch

Trachea

Rib I

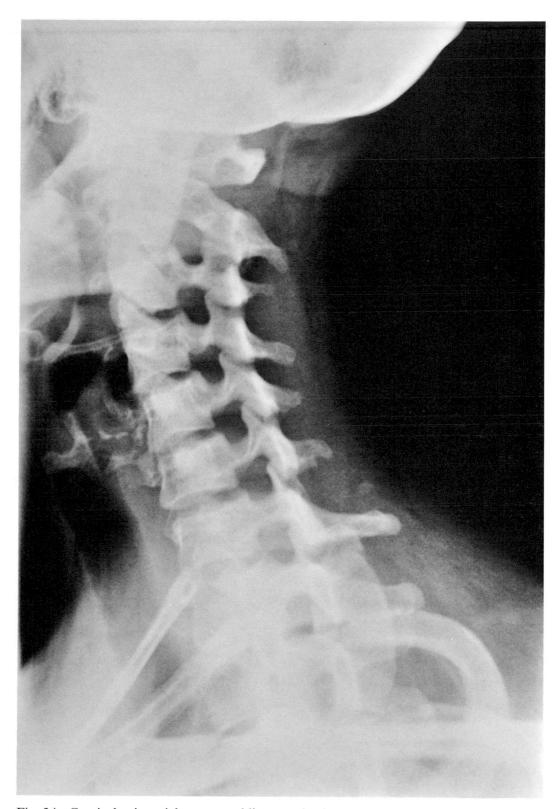

Fig. 34. Cervical spine, right antero-oblique projection

# Thoracic Spine

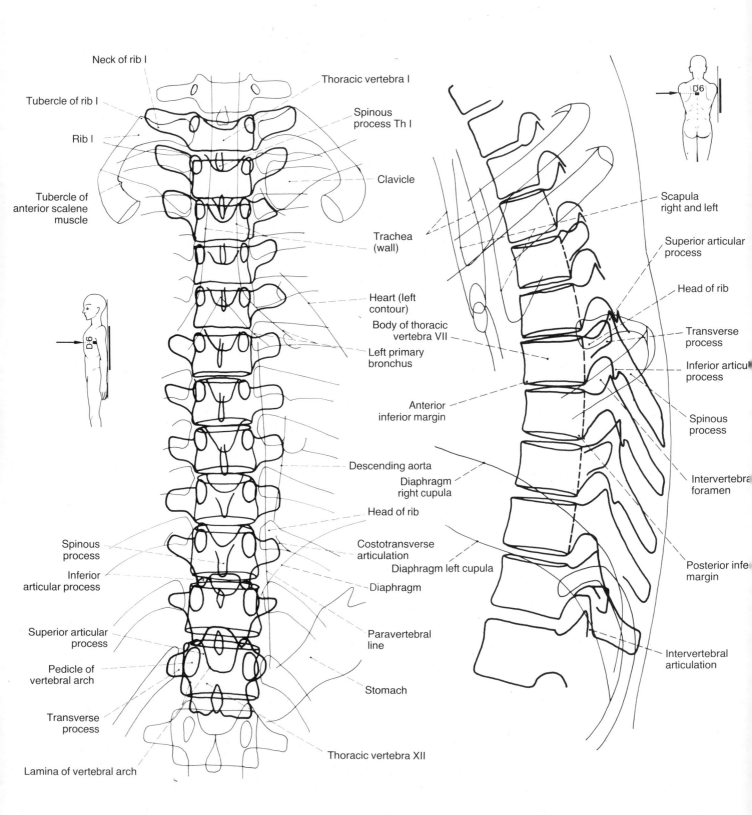

Neck of rib I

Tubercle of rib I

Rib I

Tubercle of anterior scalene muscle

Thoracic vertebra I

Spinous process Th I

Clavicle

Trachea (wall)

Heart (left contour)

Body of thoracic vertebra VII

Left primary bronchus

Anterior inferior margin

Descending aorta

Diaphragm right cupula

Head of rib

Costotransverse articulation

Diaphragm left cupula

Diaphragm

Paravertebral line

Stomach

Thoracic vertebra XII

Spinous process

Inferior articular process

Superior articular process

Pedicle of vertebral arch

Transverse process

Lamina of vertebral arch

Scapula right and left

Superior articular process

Head of rib

Transverse process

Inferior articular process

Spinous process

Intervertebral foramen

Posterior inferior margin

Intervertebral articulation

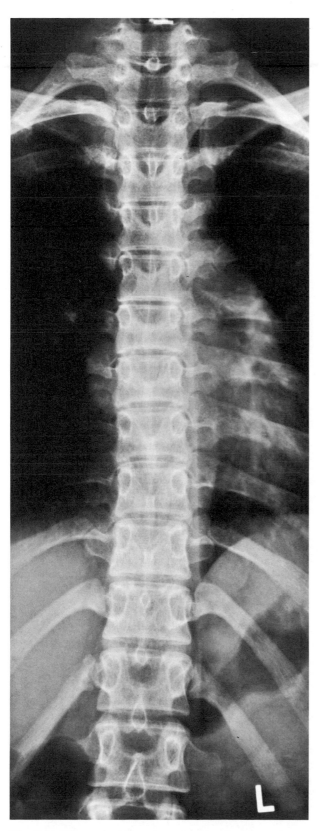

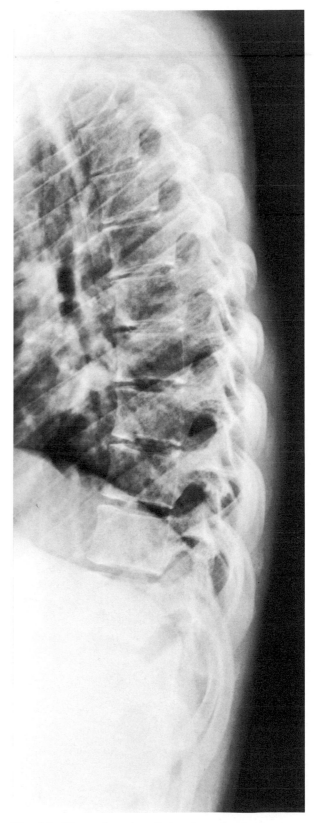

Fig. 35.  Thoracic spine (a.p. projection)     Fig. 36.  Thoracic spine (lateral projection)

# Lumbar Spine

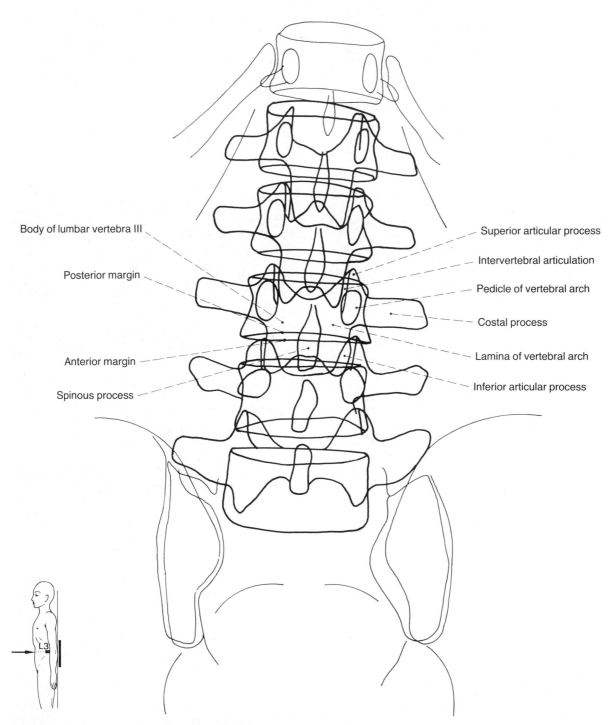

Body of lumbar vertebra III

Posterior margin

Anterior margin

Spinous process

Superior articular process

Intervertebral articulation

Pedicle of vertebral arch

Costal process

Lamina of vertebral arch

Inferior articular process

L3

(Anatomical details labeled only on the third lumbar vertebra)

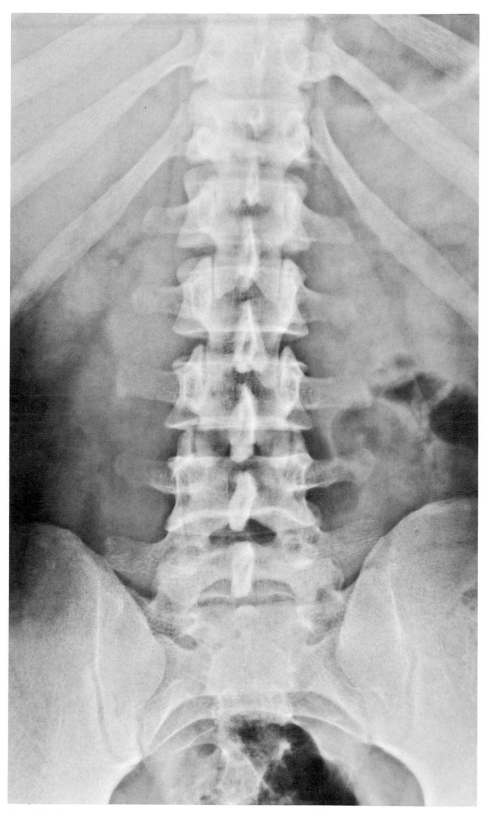

Fig. 37. Lumbar spine (a.p. projection)

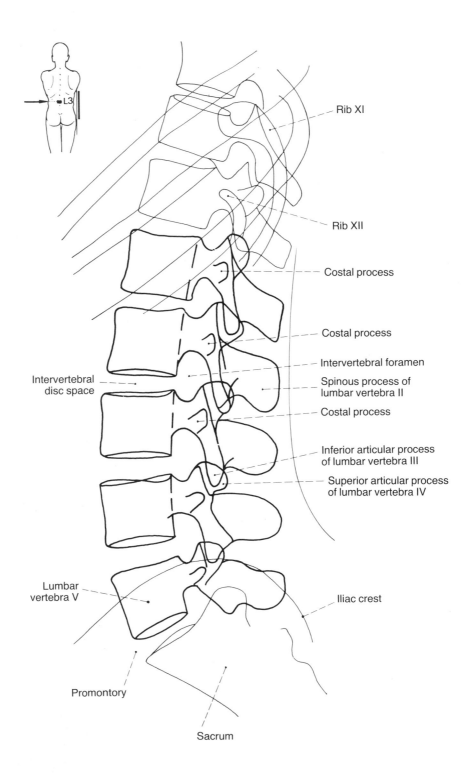

Rib XI

Rib XII

Costal process

Costal process

Intervertebral foramen

Spinous process of
lumbar vertebra II

Costal process

Inferior articular process
of lumbar vertebra III

Superior articular process
of lumbar vertebra IV

Intervertebral
disc space

Lumbar
vertebra V

Iliac crest

Promontory

Sacrum

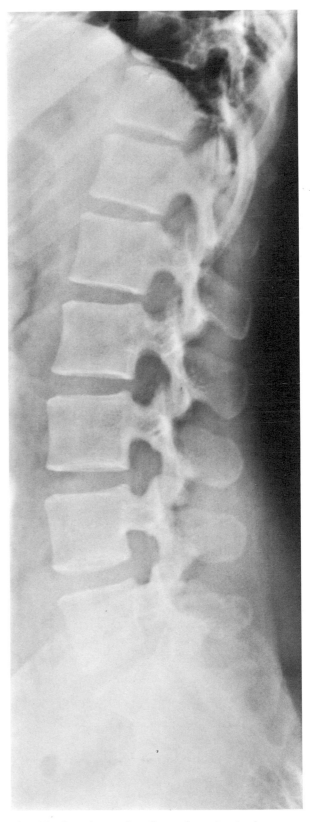

Fig. 38.  Lumbar spine (lateral projection)

# Lumbar Spine

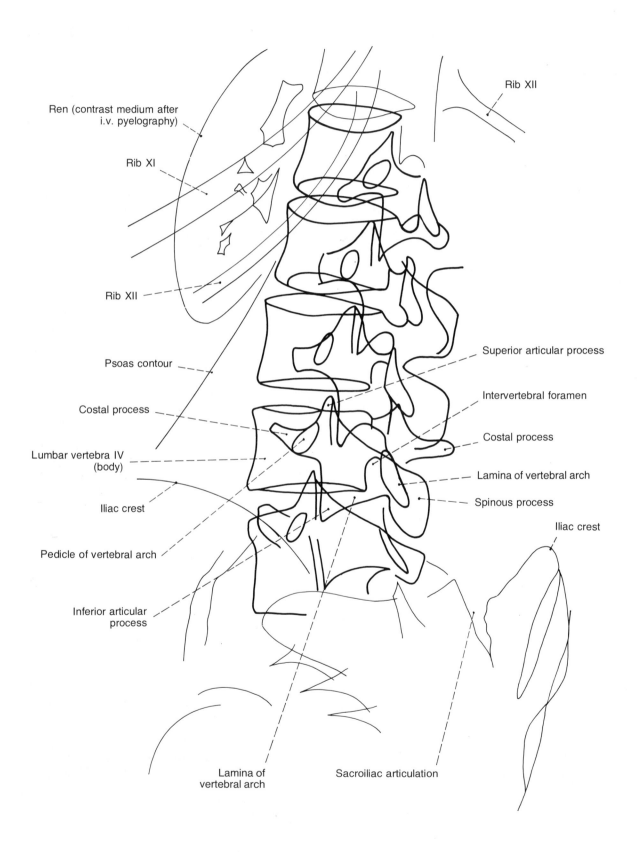

Ren (contrast medium after i.v. pyelography)

Rib XI

Rib XII

Psoas contour

Costal process

Lumbar vertebra IV (body)

Iliac crest

Pedicle of vertebral arch

Inferior articular process

Rib XII

Superior articular process

Intervertebral foramen

Costal process

Lamina of vertebral arch

Spinous process

Iliac crest

Lamina of vertebral arch

Sacroiliac articulation

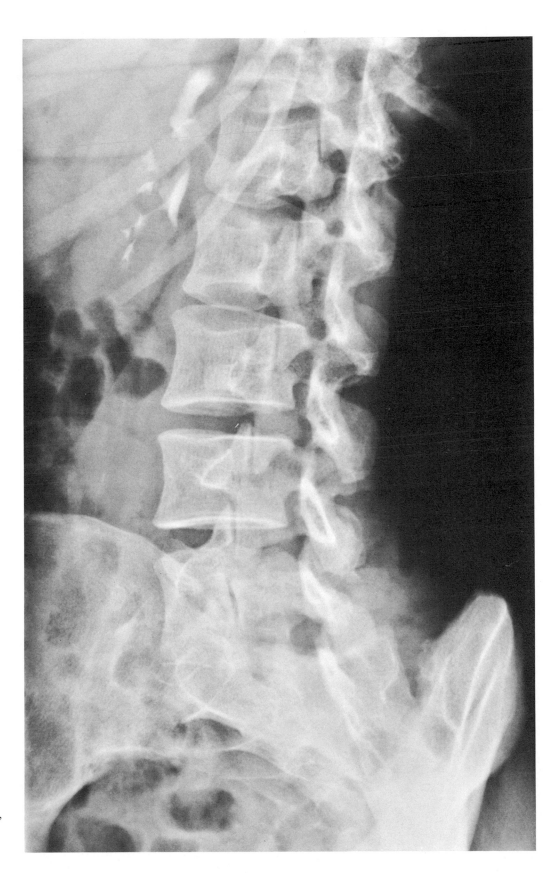

Fig. 39. Lumbar spine, right antero-oblique projection

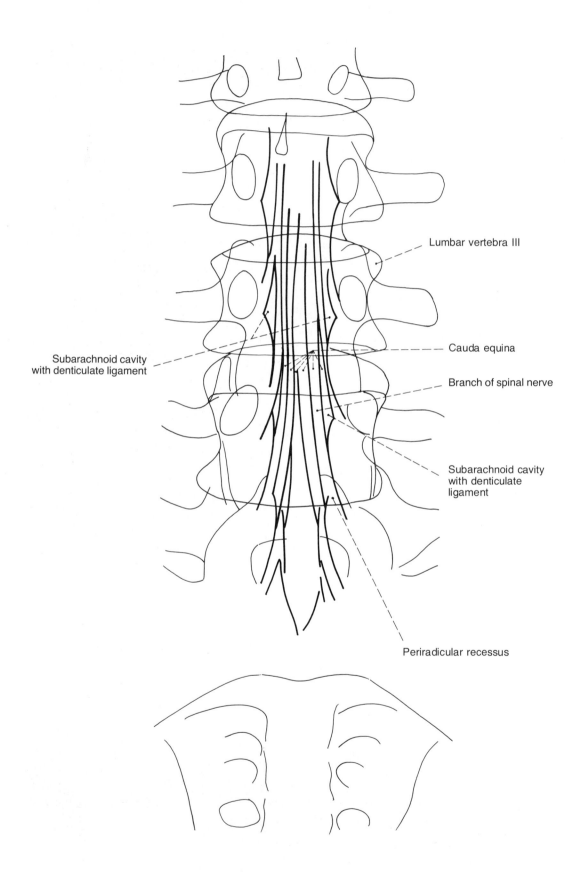

Lumbar vertebra III

Cauda equina

Branch of spinal nerve

Subarachnoid cavity
with denticulate ligament

Subarachnoid cavity
with denticulate
ligament

Periradicular recessus

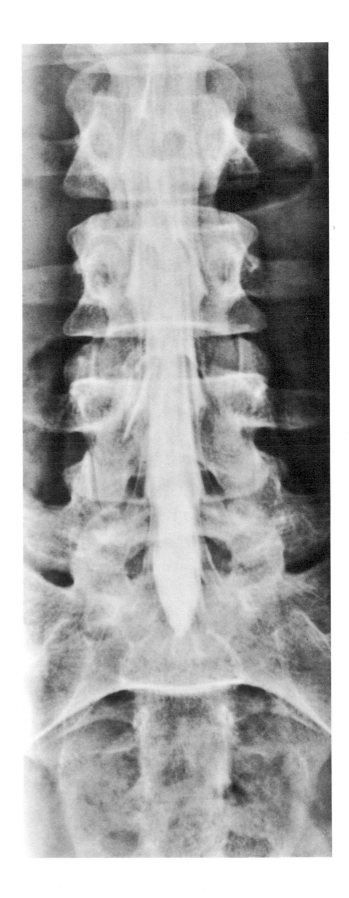

Fig. 40.  Myelography (p.a. projection)

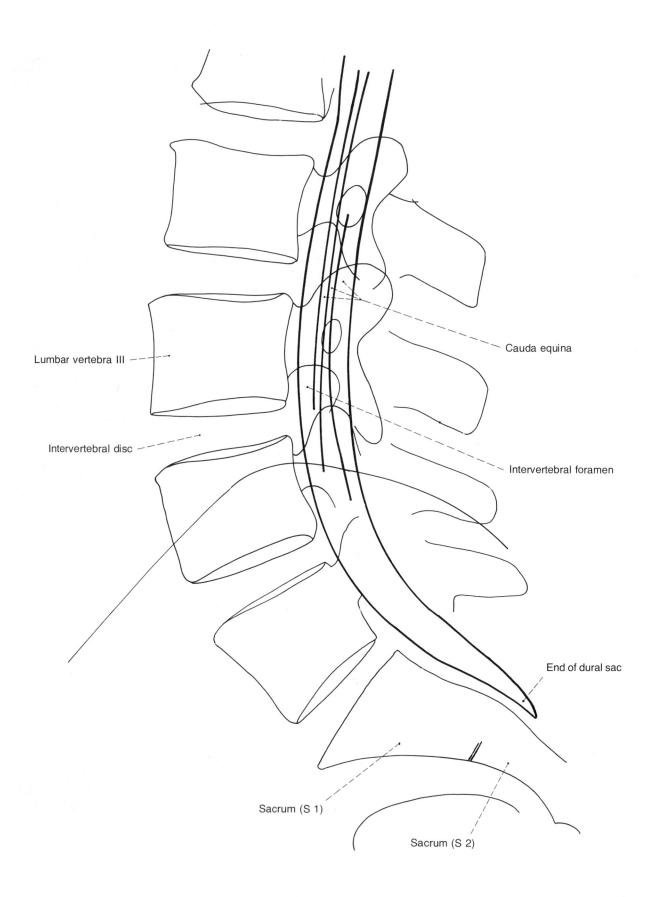

Lumbar vertebra III

Intervertebral disc

Cauda equina

Intervertebral foramen

End of dural sac

Sacrum (S 1)

Sacrum (S 2)

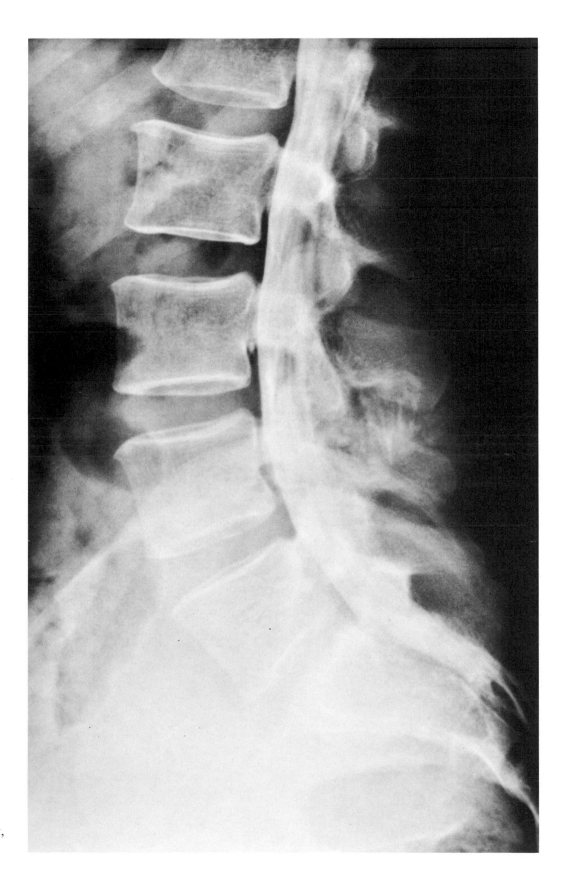

Fig. 41. Myelography,
lateral projection

# Pelvis

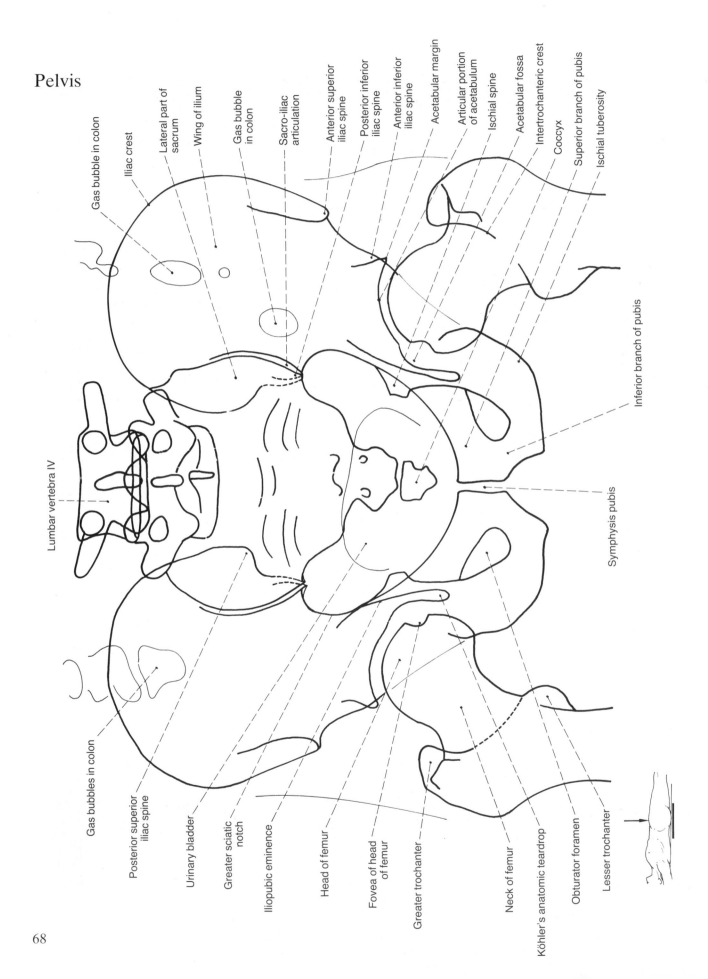

Gas bubble in colon

Iliac crest

Lateral part of sacrum

Wing of ilium

Gas bubble in colon

Sacro-iliac articulation

Anterior superior iliac spine

Posterior inferior iliac spine

Anterior inferior iliac spine

Acetabular margin

Articular portion of acetabulum

Ischial spine

Acetabular fossa

Intertrochanteric crest

Coccyx

Superior branch of pubis

Ischial tuberosity

Inferior branch of pubis

Lumbar vertebra IV

Symphysis pubis

Gas bubbles in colon

Posterior superior iliac spine

Urinary bladder

Greater sciatic notch

Iliopubic eminence

Head of femur

Fovea of head of femur

Greater trochanter

Neck of femur

Köhler's anatomic teardrop

Obturator foramen

Lesser trochanter

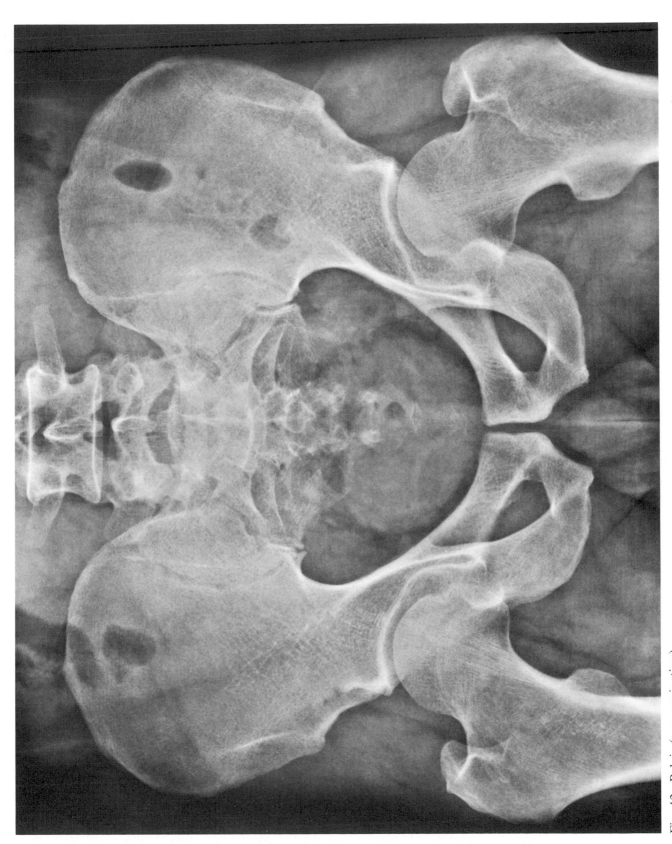

Fig. 42. Pelvis (a.p. projection)

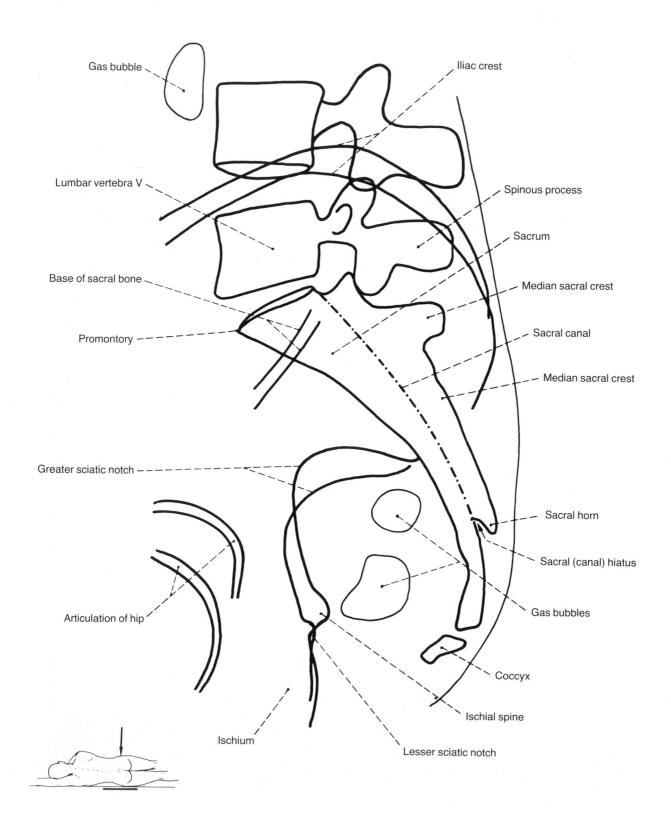

Gas bubble

Iliac crest

Lumbar vertebra V

Spinous process

Sacrum

Base of sacral bone

Median sacral crest

Promontory

Sacral canal

Median sacral crest

Greater sciatic notch

Sacral horn

Sacral (canal) hiatus

Articulation of hip

Gas bubbles

Ischium

Coccyx

Ischial spine

Lesser sciatic notch

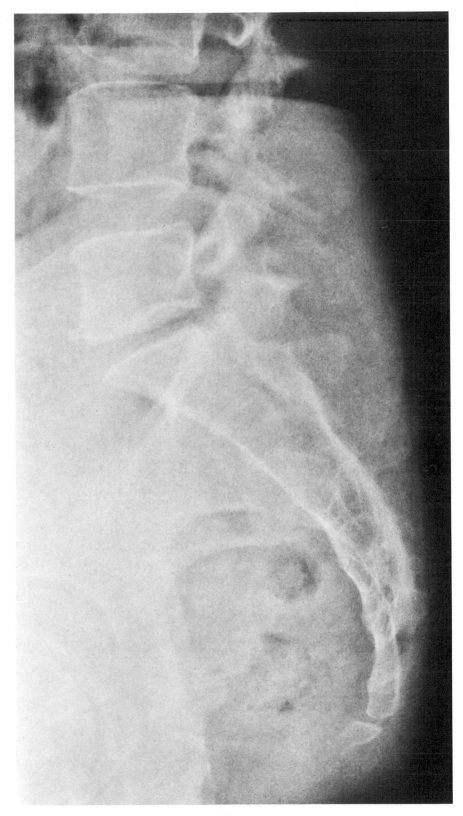

Fig. 43. Sacrum (lateral projection)

# Iliac Arteries

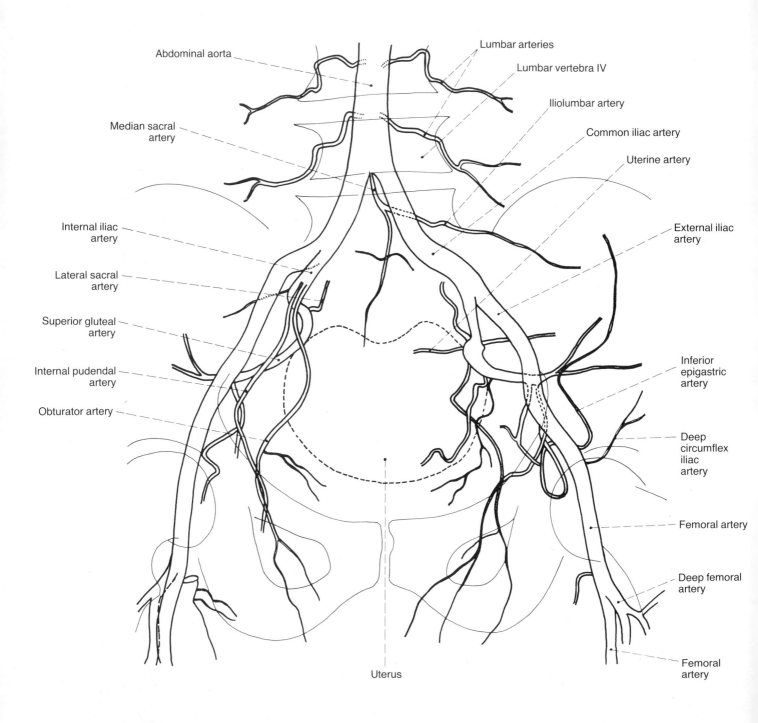

Abdominal aorta

Lumbar arteries

Lumbar vertebra IV

Median sacral artery

Iliolumbar artery

Common iliac artery

Uterine artery

Internal iliac artery

External iliac artery

Lateral sacral artery

Superior gluteal artery

Internal pudendal artery

Inferior epigastric artery

Obturator artery

Deep circumflex iliac artery

Femoral artery

Deep femoral artery

Femoral artery

Uterus

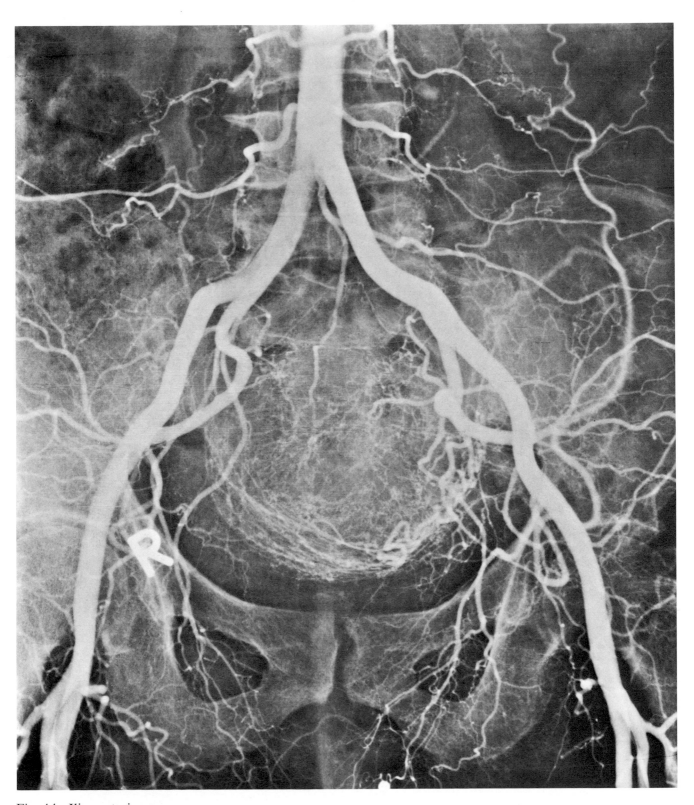

Fig. 44.  Iliac arteriogram

# Upper Extremity

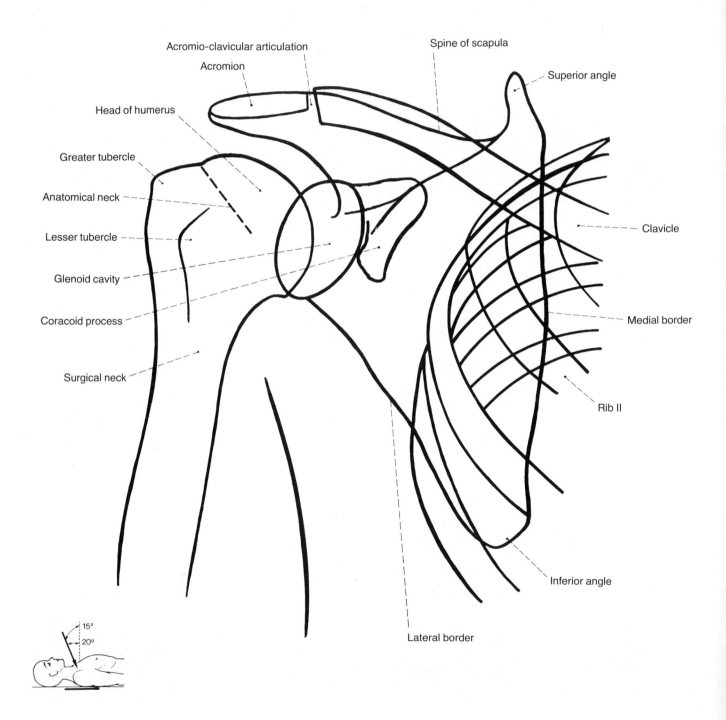

Acromio-clavicular articulation

Spine of scapula

Acromion

Superior angle

Head of humerus

Greater tubercle

Clavicle

Anatomical neck

Lesser tubercle

Glenoid cavity

Medial border

Coracoid process

Surgical neck

Rib II

Inferior angle

Lateral border

15°
20°

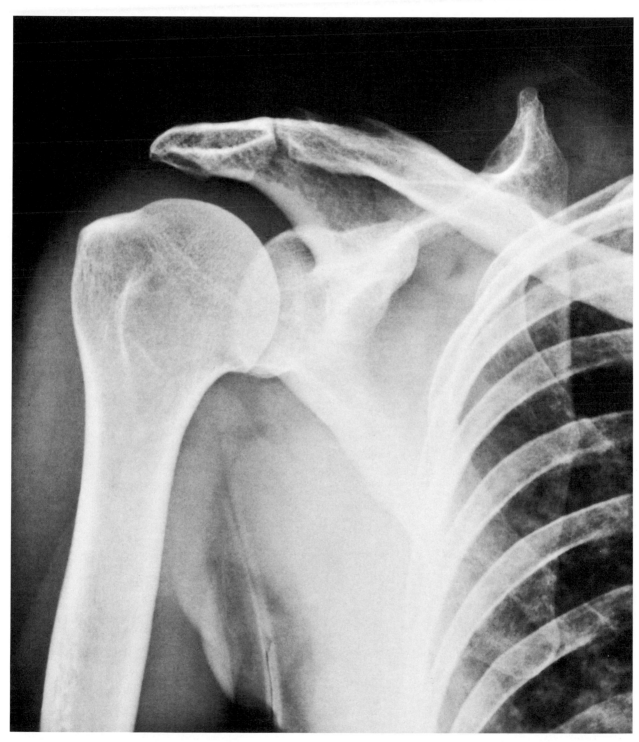

Fig. 45. Right shoulder (a.p. projection)

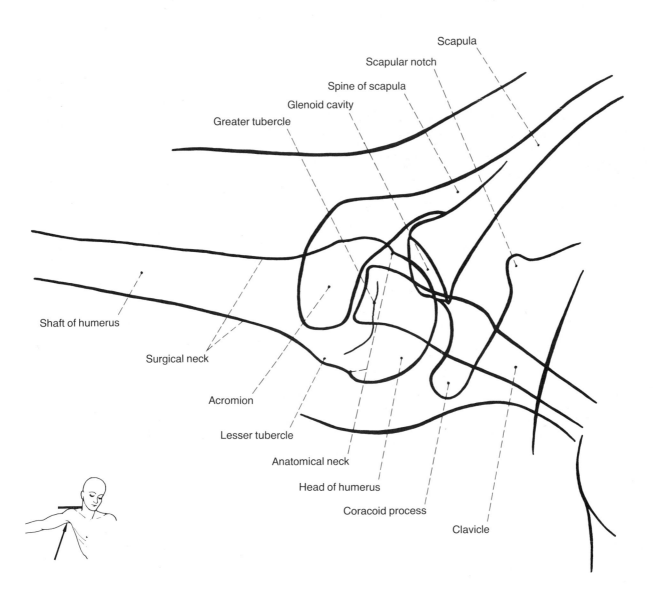

Scapula

Scapular notch

Spine of scapula

Glenoid cavity

Greater tubercle

Shaft of humerus

Surgical neck

Acromion

Lesser tubercle

Anatomical neck

Head of humerus

Coracoid process

Clavicle

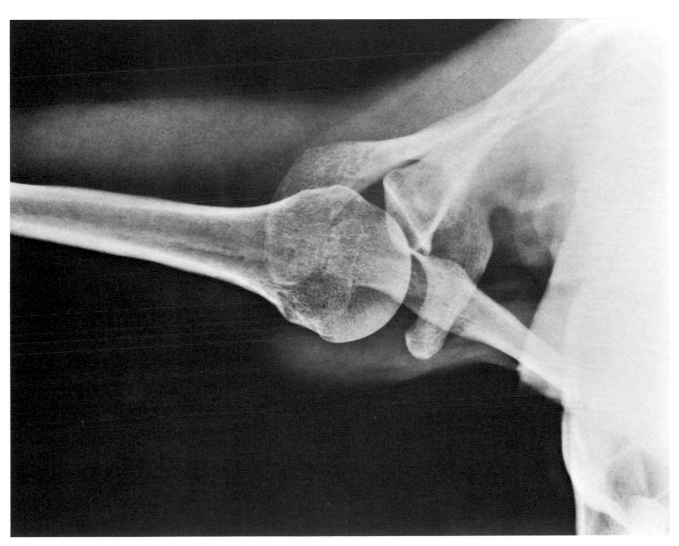

Fig. 46. Right shoulder (axial projection)

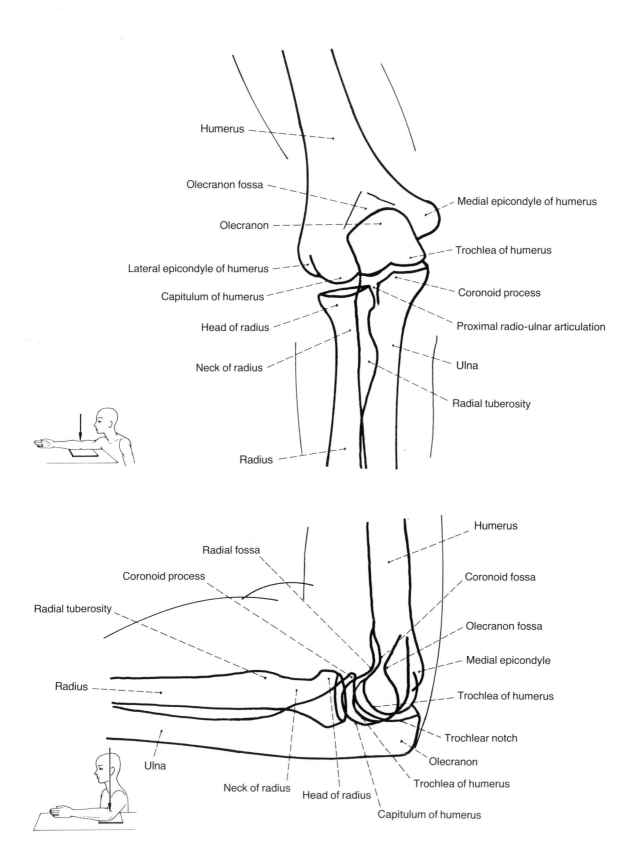

Humerus

Olecranon fossa

Olecranon

Lateral epicondyle of humerus

Capitulum of humerus

Head of radius

Neck of radius

Radius

Medial epicondyle of humerus

Trochlea of humerus

Coronoid process

Proximal radio-ulnar articulation

Ulna

Radial tuberosity

Radial fossa

Coronoid process

Radial tuberosity

Radius

Ulna

Neck of radius

Head of radius

Capitulum of humerus

Humerus

Coronoid fossa

Olecranon fossa

Medial epicondyle

Trochlea of humerus

Trochlear notch

Olecranon

Trochlea of humerus

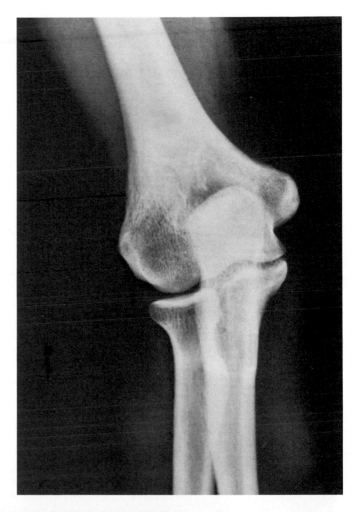

Fig. 47. Right elbow (a.p. projection)

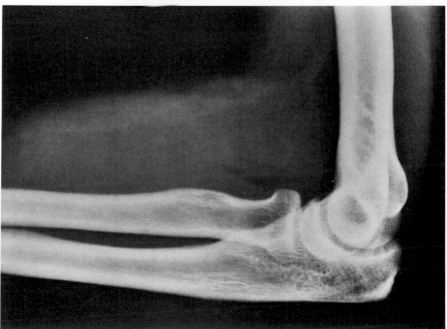

Fig. 48. Left elbow
(lateral projection)

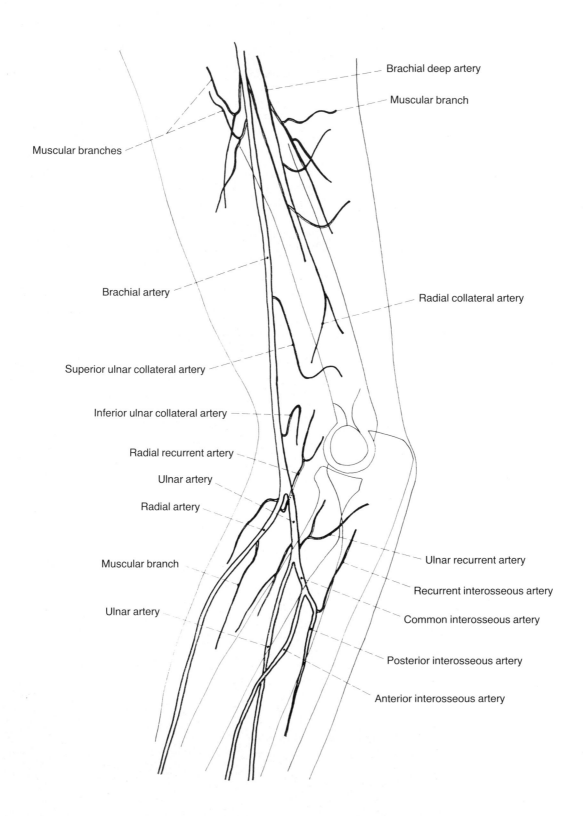

Brachial deep artery

Muscular branch

Muscular branches

Brachial artery

Radial collateral artery

Superior ulnar collateral artery

Inferior ulnar collateral artery

Radial recurrent artery

Ulnar artery

Radial artery

Muscular branch

Ulnar recurrent artery

Recurrent interosseous artery

Ulnar artery

Common interosseous artery

Posterior interosseous artery

Anterior interosseous artery

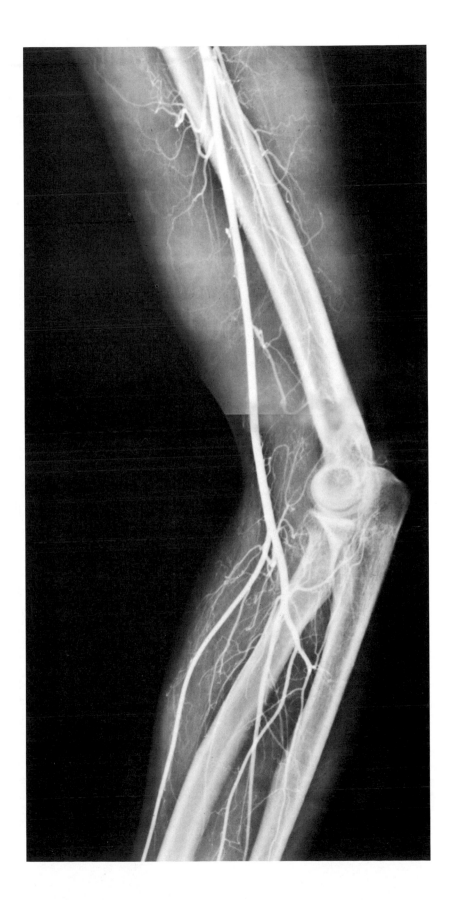

Fig. 49. Brachial arteriogram

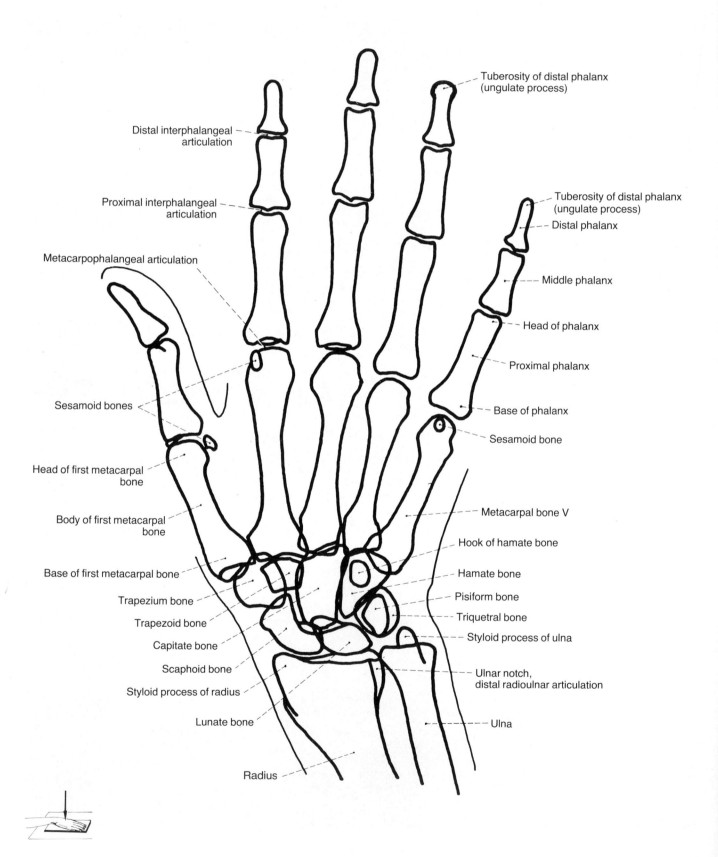

Tuberosity of distal phalanx (ungulate process)

Distal interphalangeal articulation

Proximal interphalangeal articulation

Metacarpophalangeal articulation

Sesamoid bones

Head of first metacarpal bone

Body of first metacarpal bone

Base of first metacarpal bone

Trapezium bone

Trapezoid bone

Capitate bone

Scaphoid bone

Styloid process of radius

Lunate bone

Radius

Tuberosity of distal phalanx (ungulate process)

Distal phalanx

Middle phalanx

Head of phalanx

Proximal phalanx

Base of phalanx

Sesamoid bone

Metacarpal bone V

Hook of hamate bone

Hamate bone

Pisiform bone

Triquetral bone

Styloid process of ulna

Ulnar notch, distal radioulnar articulation

Ulna

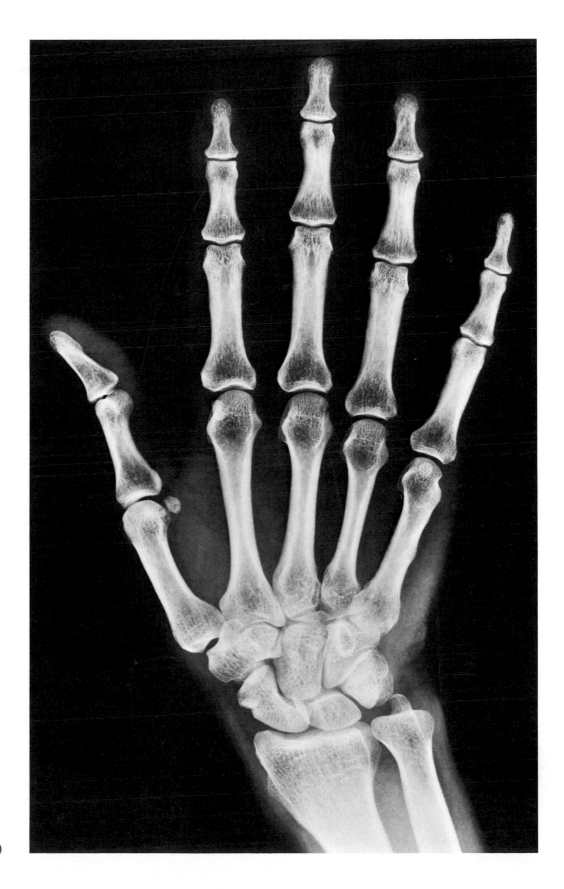

Fig. 50. Right hand
(dorsovolar projection)

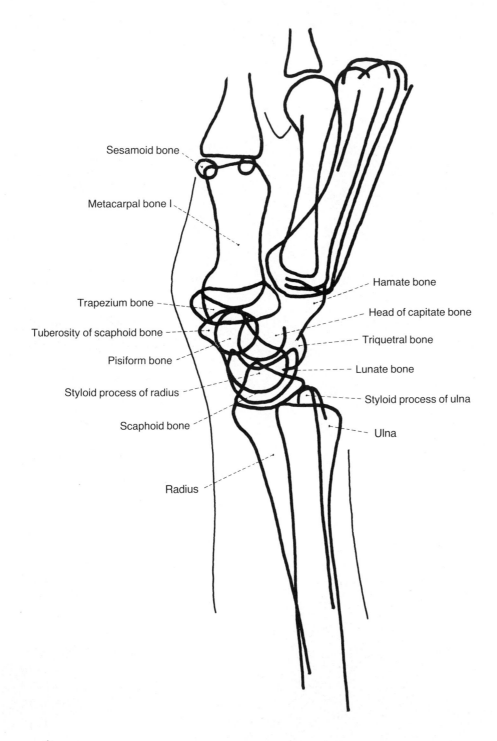

Sesamoid bone

Metacarpal bone I

Hamate bone

Trapezium bone

Head of capitate bone

Tuberosity of scaphoid bone

Triquetral bone

Pisiform bone

Lunate bone

Styloid process of radius

Styloid process of ulna

Scaphoid bone

Ulna

Radius

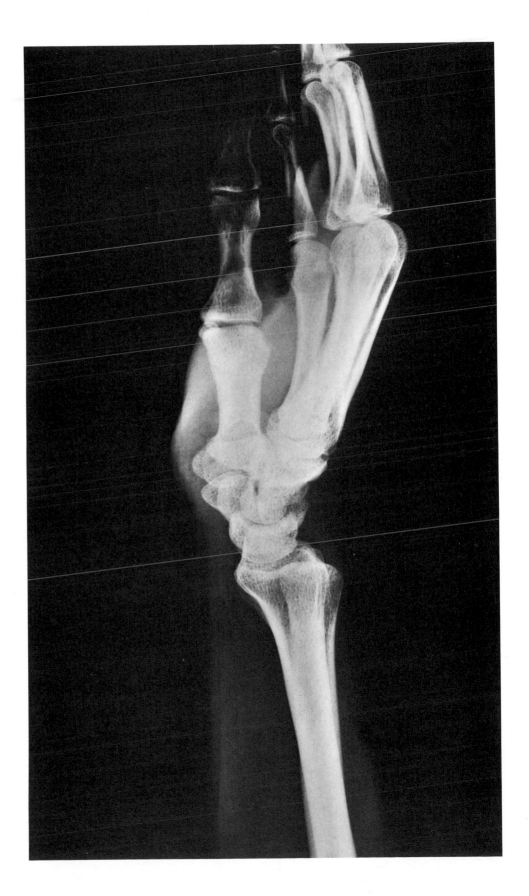

Fig. 51. Right hand
(lateral projection)

# Hand

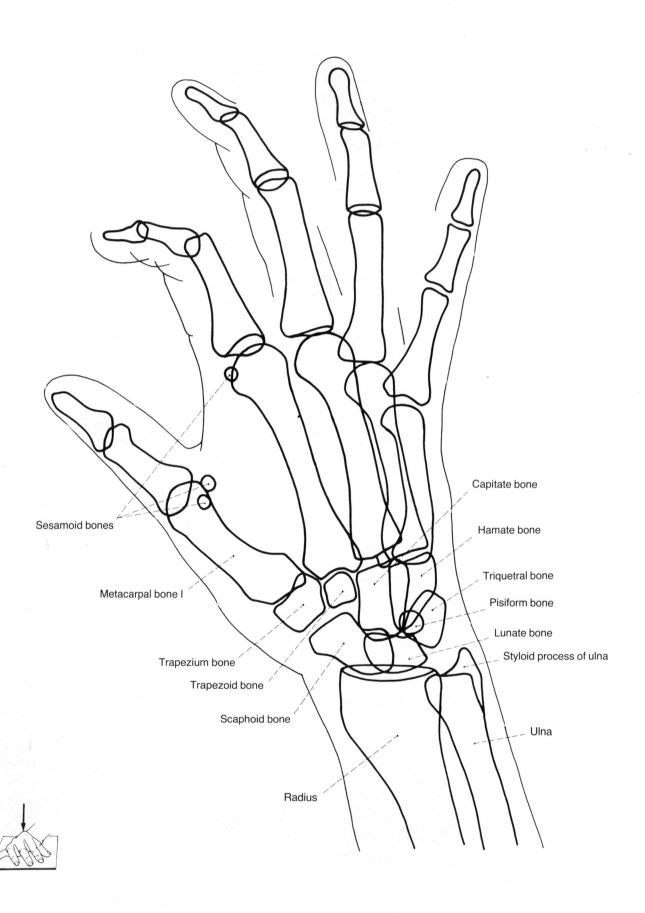

Sesamoid bones

Capitate bone

Hamate bone

Triquetral bone

Pisiform bone

Lunate bone

Styloid process of ulna

Metacarpal bone I

Trapezium bone

Trapezoid bone

Scaphoid bone

Ulna

Radius

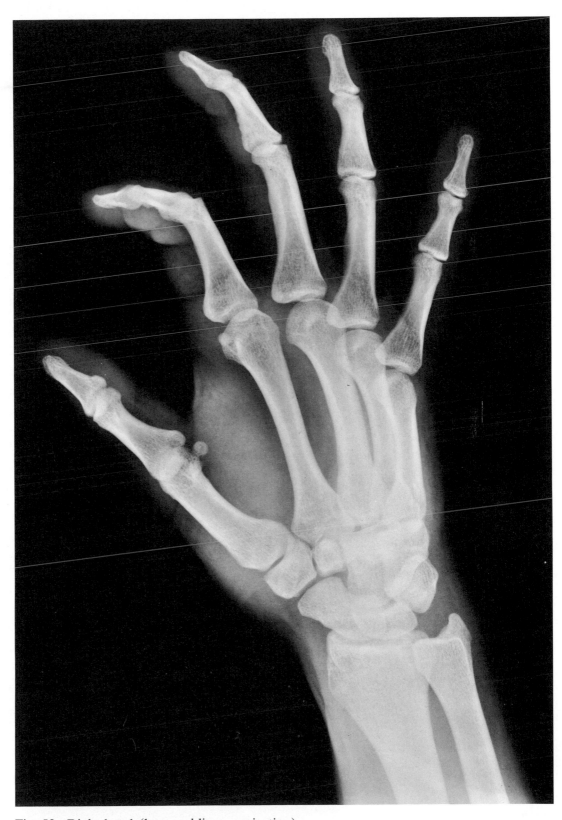

Fig. 52. Right hand (latero-oblique projection)

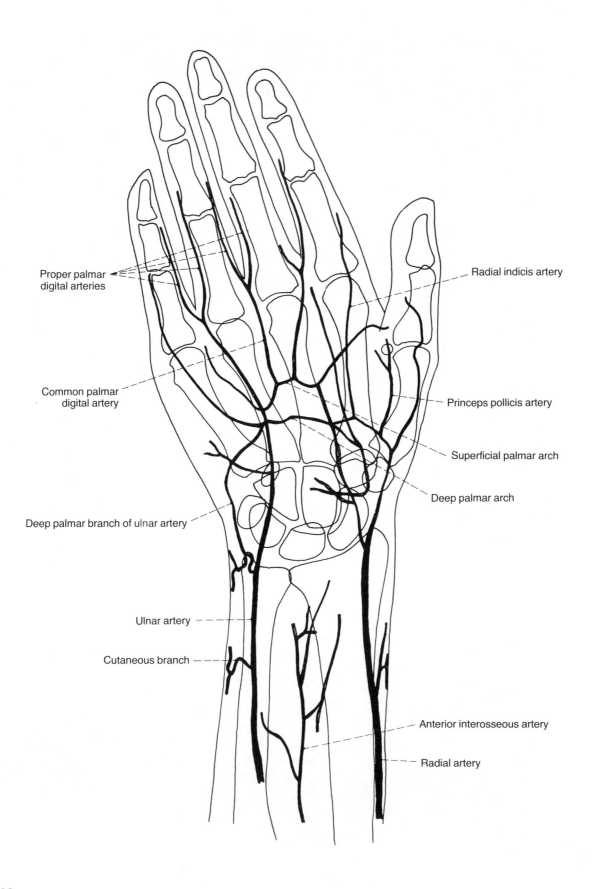

Proper palmar
digital arteries

Radial indicis artery

Common palmar
digital artery

Princeps pollicis artery

Superficial palmar arch

Deep palmar arch

Deep palmar branch of ulnar artery

Ulnar artery

Cutaneous branch

Anterior interosseous artery

Radial artery

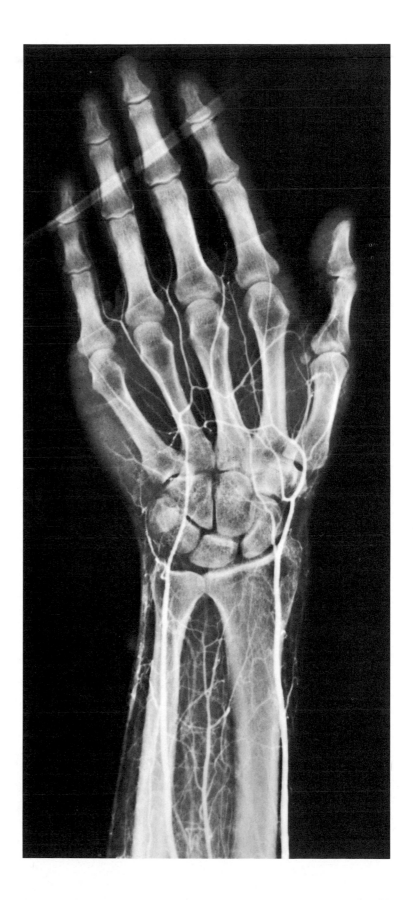

Fig. 53. Hand arteriogram

# Lower Extremity

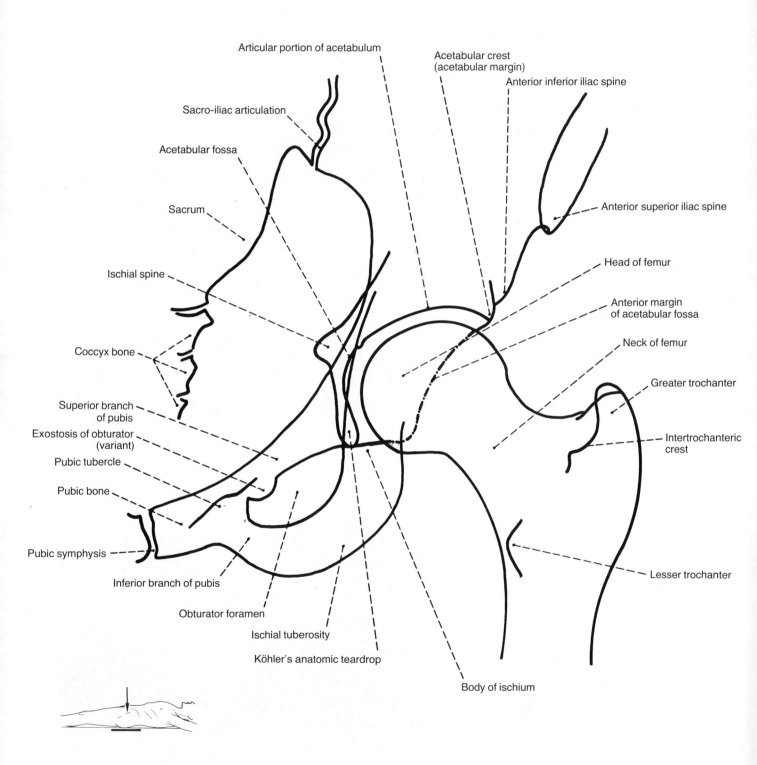

Articular portion of acetabulum

Acetabular crest (acetabular margin)

Anterior inferior iliac spine

Sacro-iliac articulation

Acetabular fossa

Sacrum

Anterior superior iliac spine

Ischial spine

Head of femur

Anterior margin of acetabular fossa

Coccyx bone

Neck of femur

Superior branch of pubis

Greater trochanter

Exostosis of obturator (variant)

Intertrochanteric crest

Pubic tubercle

Pubic bone

Pubic symphysis

Lesser trochanter

Inferior branch of pubis

Obturator foramen

Ischial tuberosity

Köhler's anatomic teardrop

Body of ischium

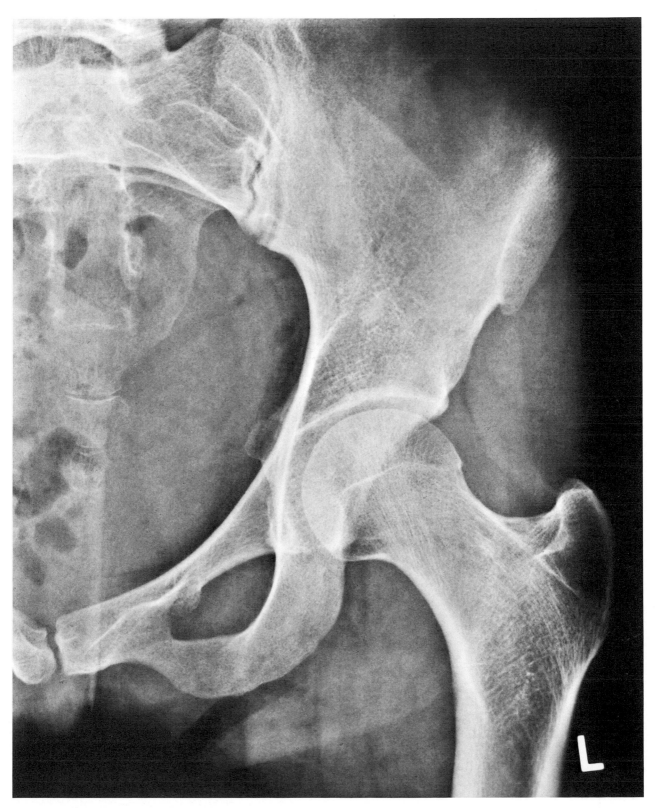

Fig. 54. Hip joint (a.p. projection)

# Hip Joint

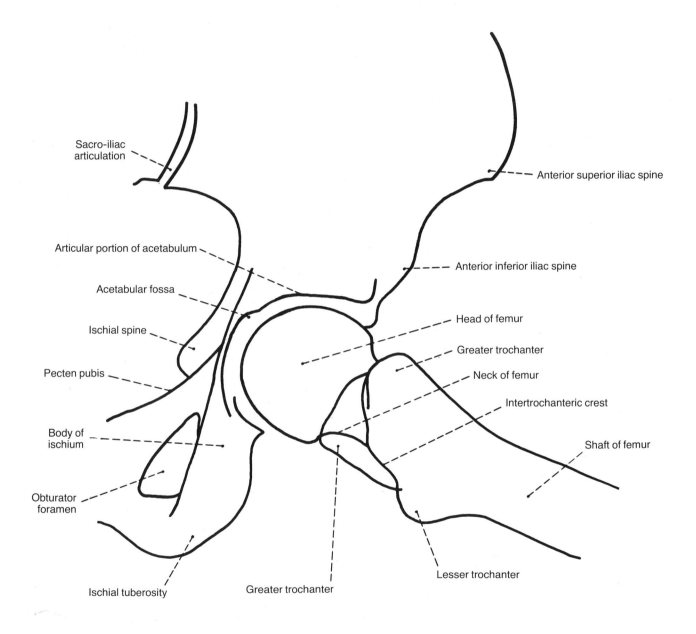

Sacro-iliac articulation

Articular portion of acetabulum

Acetabular fossa

Ischial spine

Pecten pubis

Body of ischium

Obturator foramen

Ischial tuberosity

Greater trochanter

Anterior superior iliac spine

Anterior inferior iliac spine

Head of femur

Greater trochanter

Neck of femur

Intertrochanteric crest

Shaft of femur

Lesser trochanter

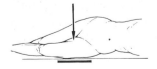

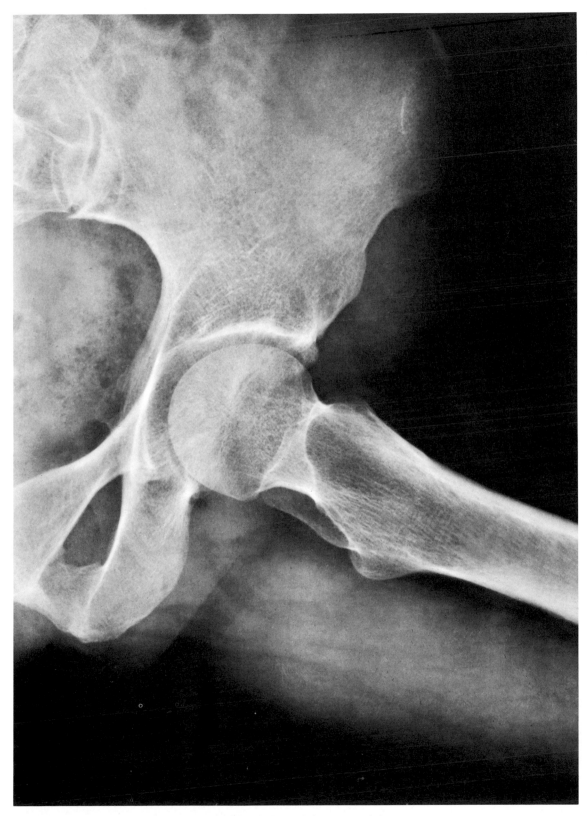

Fig. 55. Left hip joint with leg laterally abducted (Lauenstein)

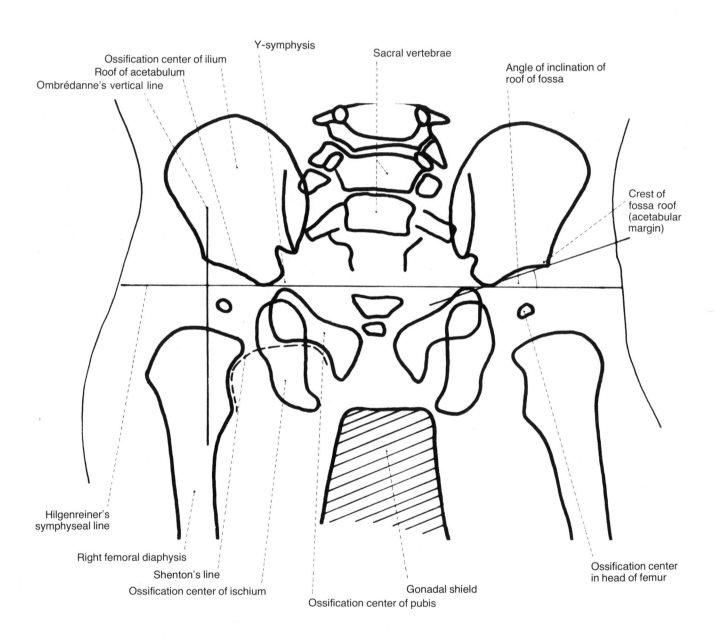

Ossification center of ilium
Roof of acetabulum
Ombrédanne's vertical line

Y-symphysis

Sacral vertebrae

Angle of inclination of
roof of fossa

Crest of
fossa roof
(acetabular
margin)

Hilgenreiner's
symphyseal line

Right femoral diaphysis

Shenton's line

Ossification center of ischium

Ossification center of pubis

Gonadal shield

Ossification center
in head of femur

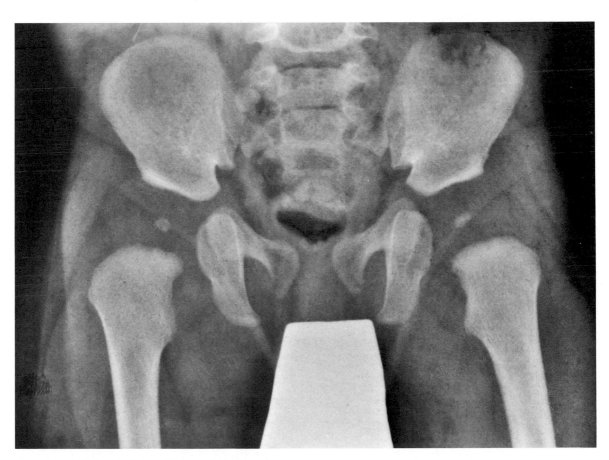

Fig. 56. Child's hip joint (7-month-old boy)

# Knee Joint

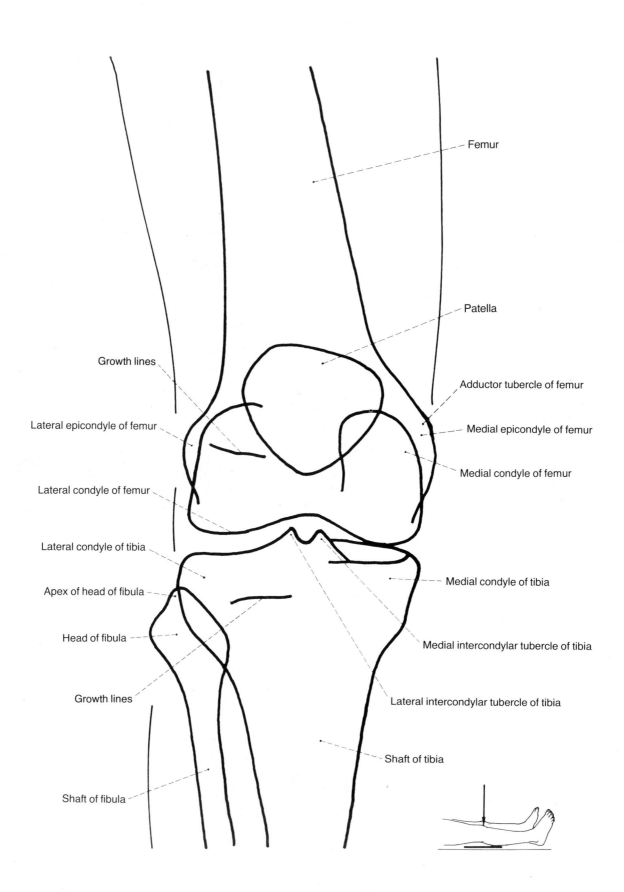

Femur

Patella

Growth lines

Adductor tubercle of femur

Lateral epicondyle of femur

Medial epicondyle of femur

Medial condyle of femur

Lateral condyle of femur

Lateral condyle of tibia

Medial condyle of tibia

Apex of head of fibula

Head of fibula

Medial intercondylar tubercle of tibia

Growth lines

Lateral intercondylar tubercle of tibia

Shaft of tibia

Shaft of fibula

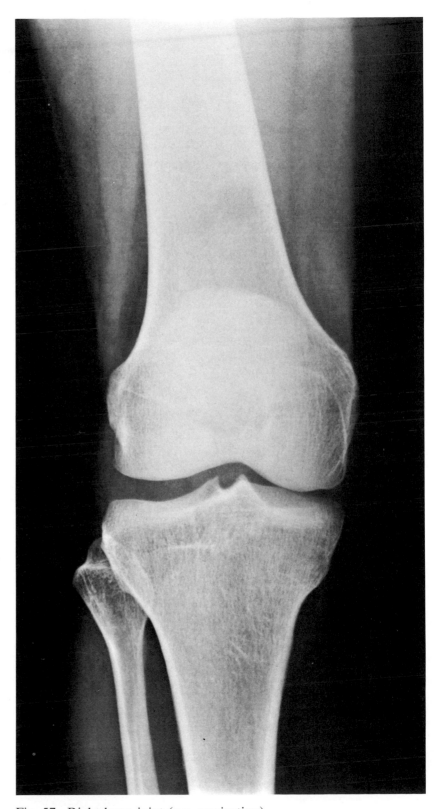

Fig. 57. Right knee joint (a.p. projection)

# Knee Joint

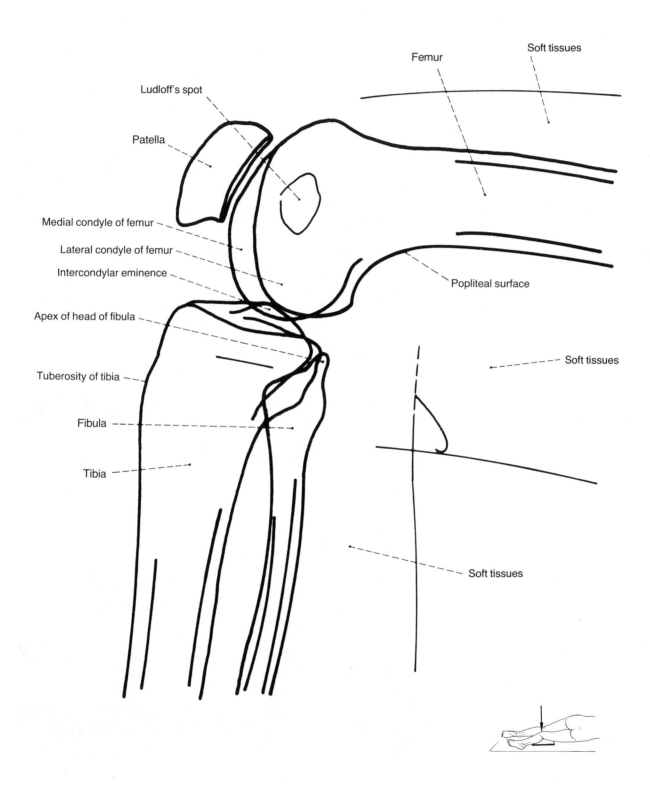

Femur

Soft tissues

Ludloff's spot

Patella

Medial condyle of femur

Lateral condyle of femur

Intercondylar eminence

Apex of head of fibula

Tuberosity of tibia

Fibula

Tibia

Popliteal surface

Soft tissues

Soft tissues

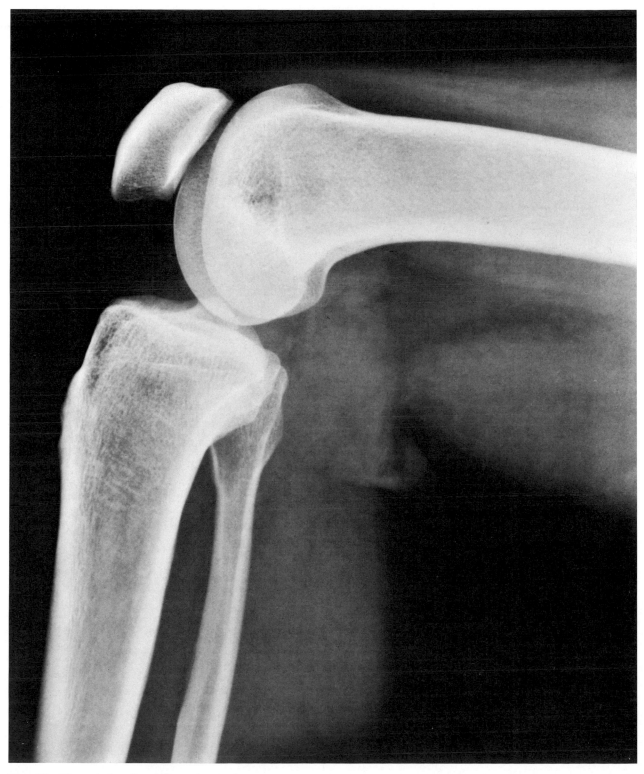

Fig. 58. Knee joint (lateral projection)

# Knee Joint

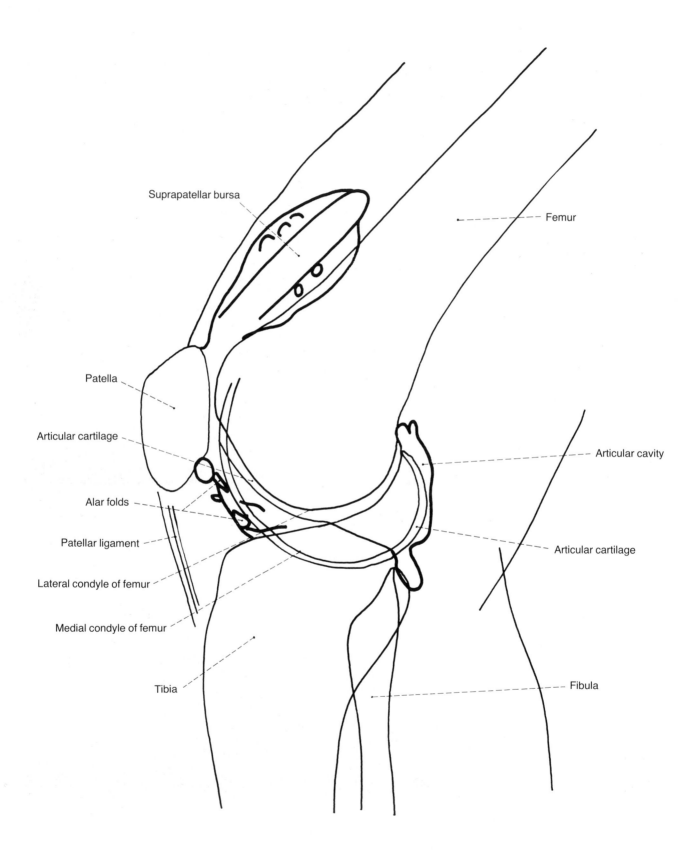

Suprapatellar bursa

Femur

Patella

Articular cartilage

Articular cavity

Alar folds

Patellar ligament

Articular cartilage

Lateral condyle of femur

Medial condyle of femur

Tibia

Fibula

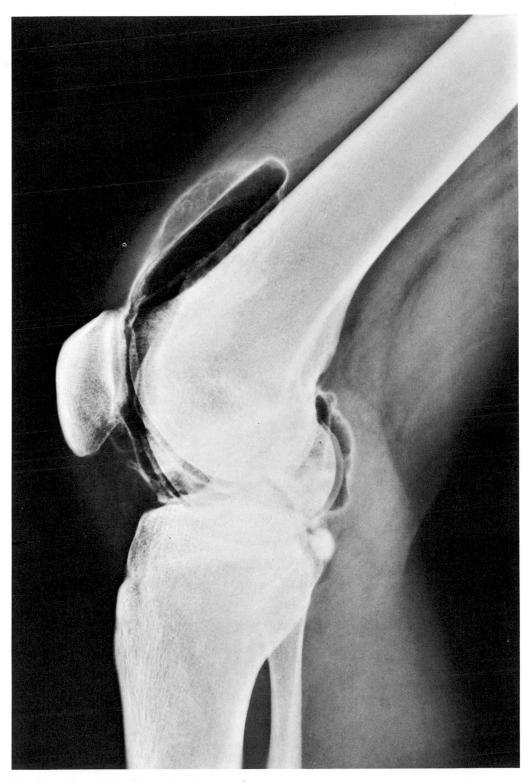

Fig. 59. Knee joint (lateral arthrogram)

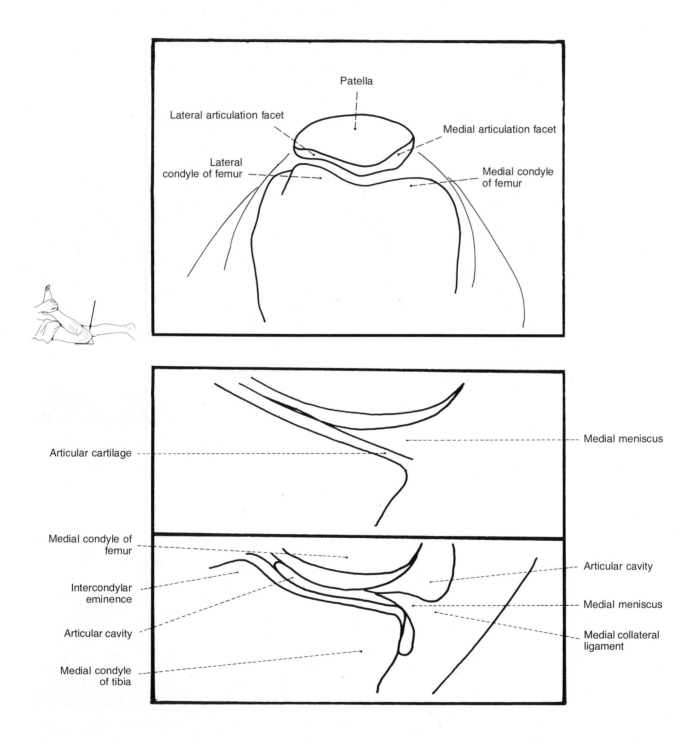

Patella

Lateral articulation facet

Medial articulation facet

Lateral condyle of femur

Medial condyle of femur

Articular cartilage

Medial meniscus

Medial condyle of femur

Articular cavity

Intercondylar eminence

Medial meniscus

Articular cavity

Medial collateral ligament

Medial condyle of tibia

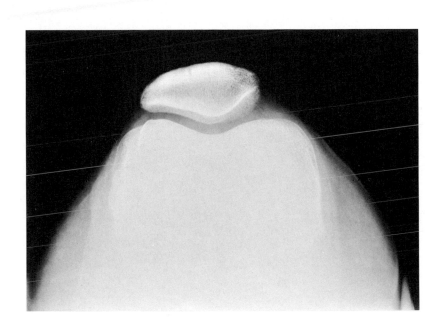

Fig. 60. Patella, axial projection

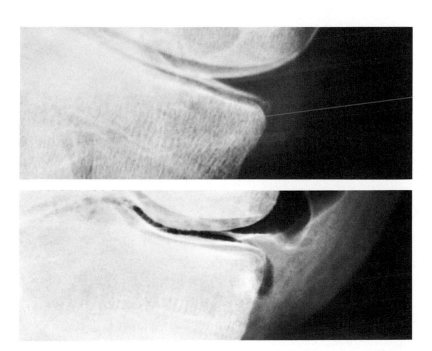

Fig. 61. Knee joint, arthrography, a.p. projection (reconnaissance radiograph from the medial meniscus)

# Knee Joint

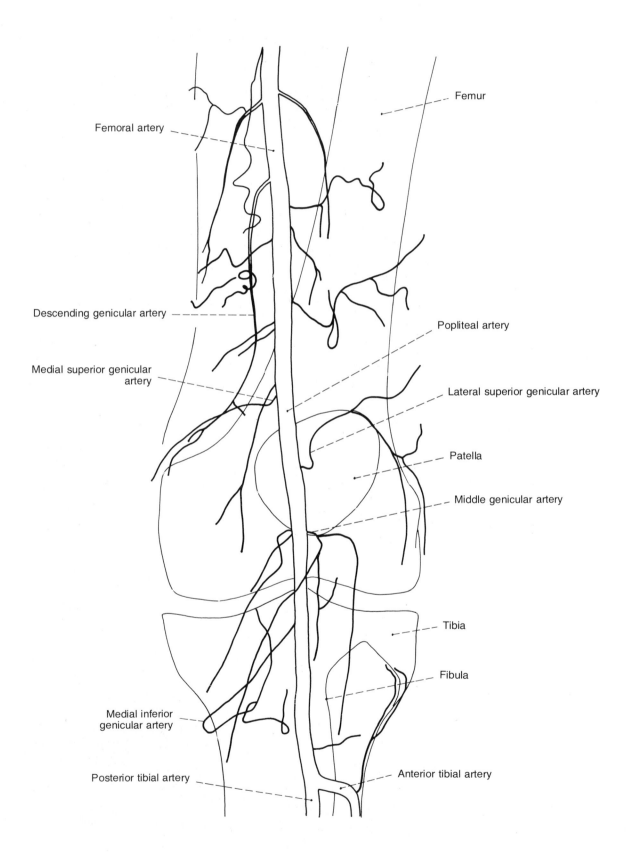

Femur

Femoral artery

Descending genicular artery

Popliteal artery

Medial superior genicular artery

Lateral superior genicular artery

Patella

Middle genicular artery

Tibia

Fibula

Medial inferior genicular artery

Posterior tibial artery

Anterior tibial artery

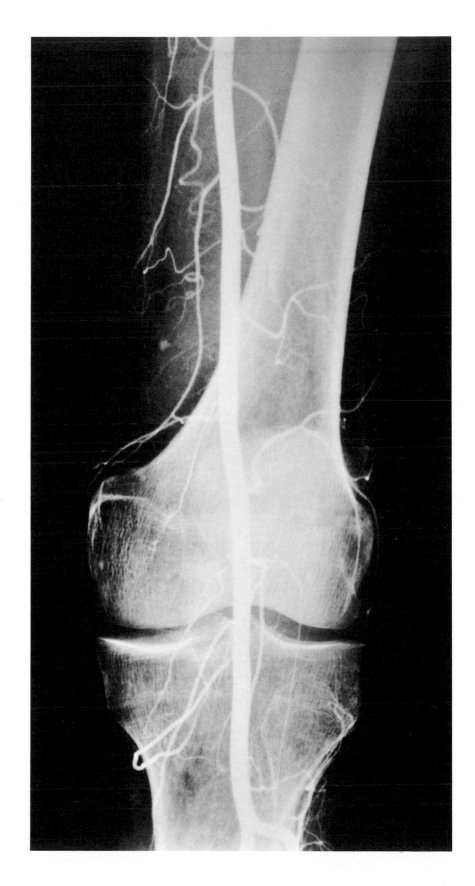

Fig. 62. Left knee joint, arteriogram
(a.p. projection)

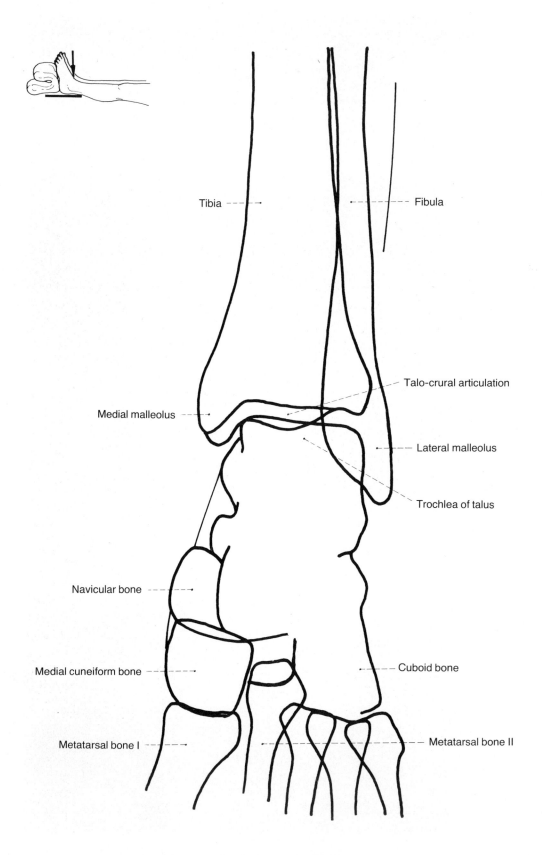

Tibia

Fibula

Talo-crural articulation

Medial malleolus

Lateral malleolus

Trochlea of talus

Navicular bone

Medial cuneiform bone

Cuboid bone

Metatarsal bone I

Metatarsal bone II

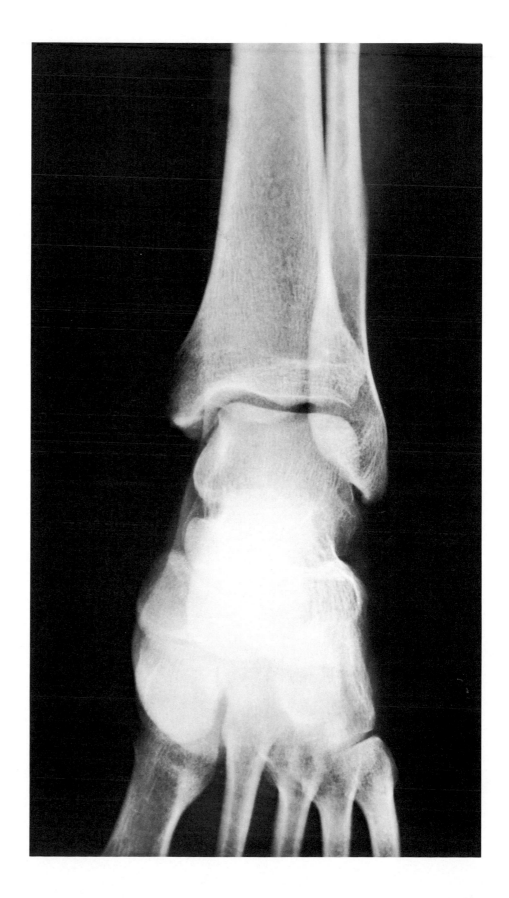

Fig. 63. Left ankle
(a.p. projection)

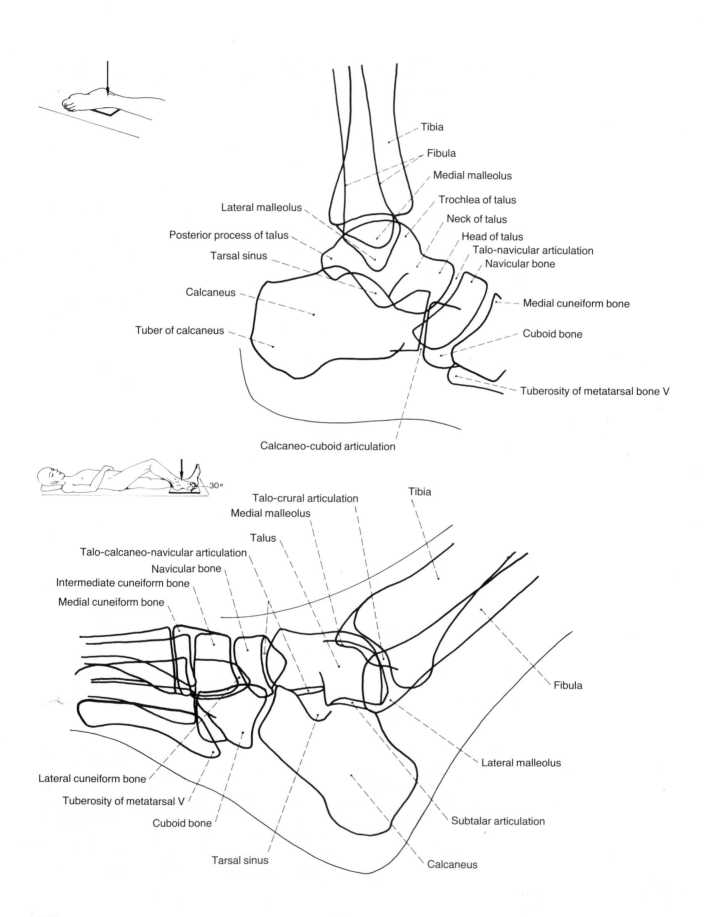

Tibia

Fibula

Medial malleolus

Trochlea of talus

Neck of talus

Lateral malleolus

Head of talus

Posterior process of talus

Talo-navicular articulation

Navicular bone

Tarsal sinus

Calcaneus

Medial cuneiform bone

Tuber of calcaneus

Cuboid bone

Tuberosity of metatarsal bone V

Calcaneo-cuboid articulation

30°

Talo-crural articulation

Medial malleolus

Tibia

Talus

Talo-calcaneo-navicular articulation

Navicular bone

Intermediate cuneiform bone

Medial cuneiform bone

Fibula

Lateral malleolus

Lateral cuneiform bone

Tuberosity of metatarsal V

Cuboid bone

Subtalar articulation

Tarsal sinus

Calcaneus

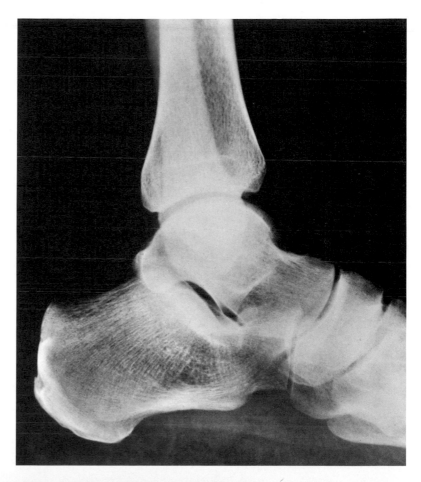

Fig. 64. Left ankle (lateral projection)

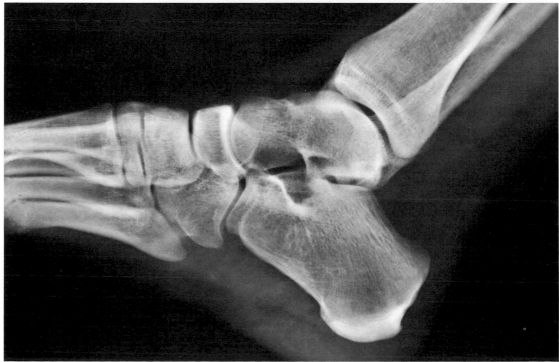

Fig. 65.
Right ankle
(oblique
projection)

# Foot

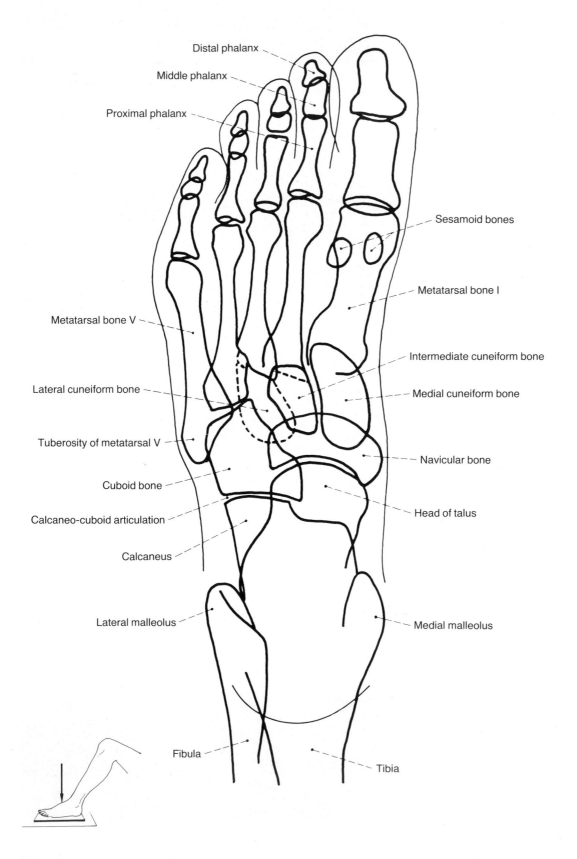

Distal phalanx

Middle phalanx

Proximal phalanx

Sesamoid bones

Metatarsal bone I

Metatarsal bone V

Intermediate cuneiform bone

Lateral cuneiform bone

Medial cuneiform bone

Tuberosity of metatarsal V

Navicular bone

Cuboid bone

Calcaneo-cuboid articulation

Head of talus

Calcaneus

Lateral malleolus

Medial malleolus

Fibula

Tibia

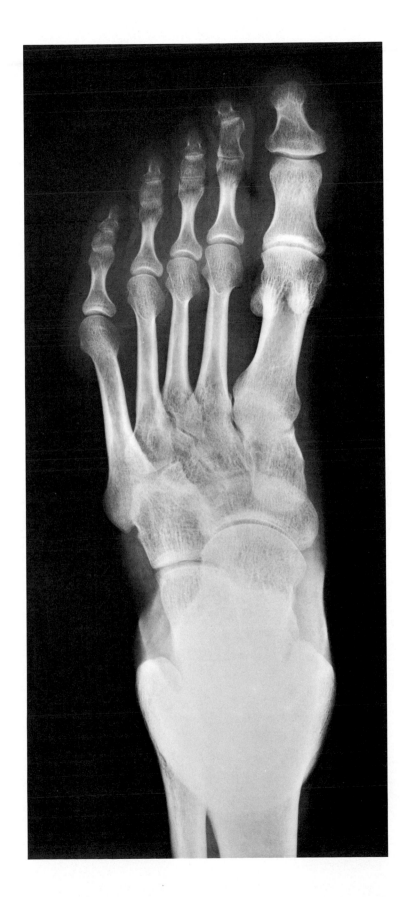

Fig. 66. Left foot (dorsoplantar projection)

# Foot

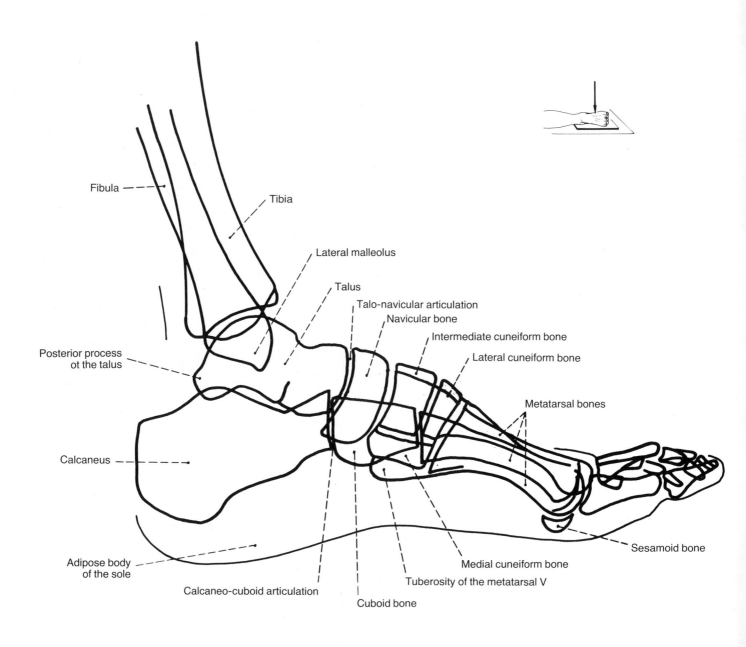

Fibula

Tibia

Lateral malleolus

Talus

Talo-navicular articulation

Navicular bone

Intermediate cuneiform bone

Lateral cuneiform bone

Metatarsal bones

Posterior process
ot the talus

Calcaneus

Sesamoid bone

Adipose body
of the sole

Medial cuneiform bone

Calcaneo-cuboid articulation

Tuberosity of the metatarsal V

Cuboid bone

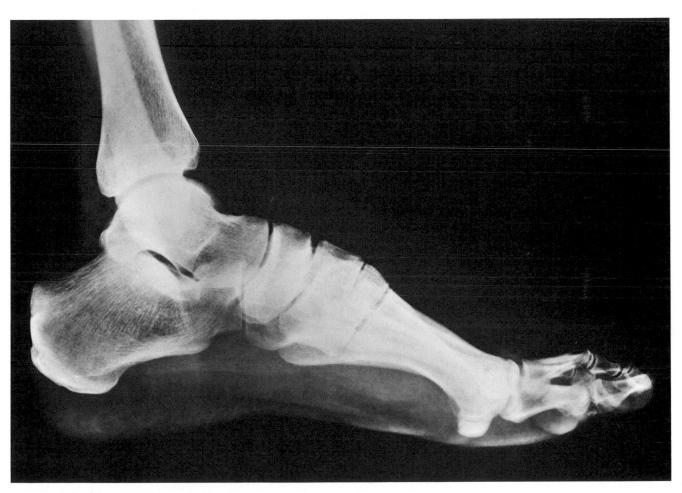

Fig. 67. Left foot (lateral projection)

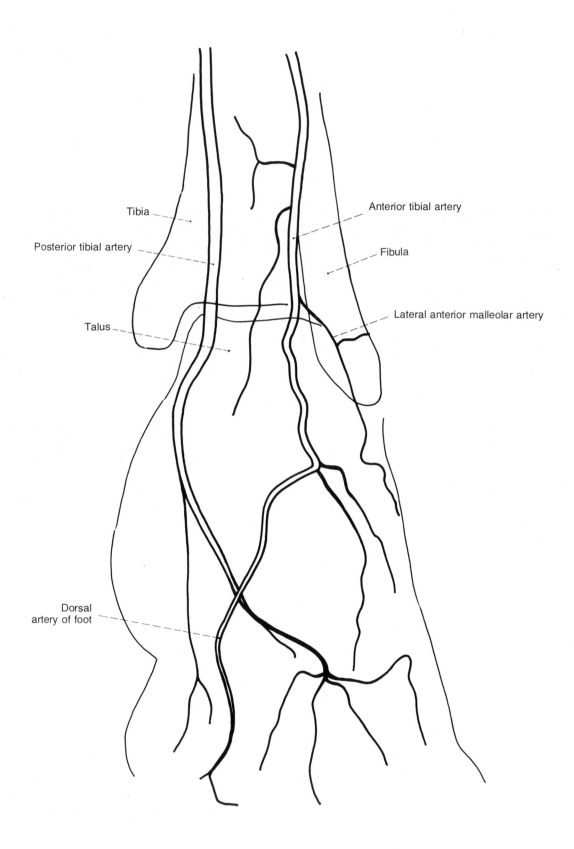

Tibia

Anterior tibial artery

Posterior tibial artery

Fibula

Talus

Lateral anterior malleolar artery

Dorsal
artery of foot

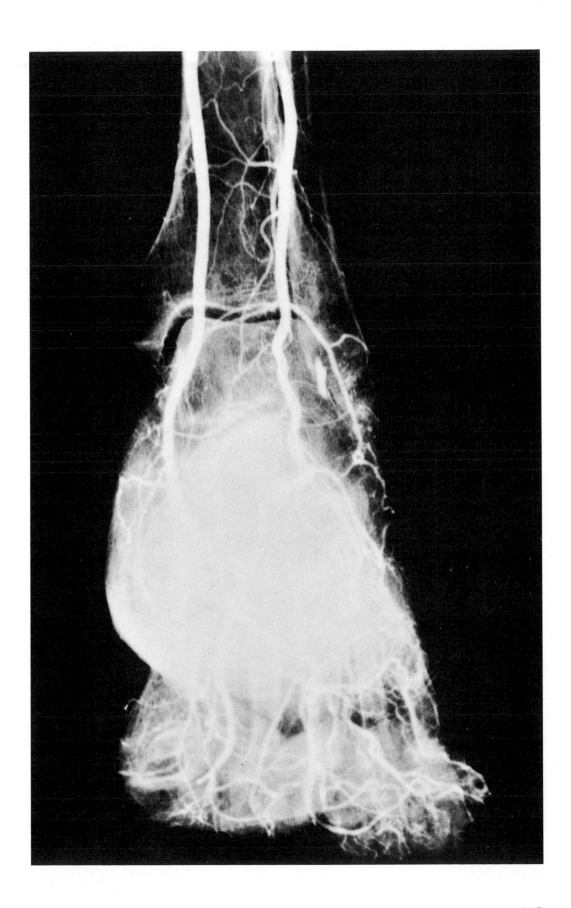

Fig. 68.
Left ankle joint,
angiography
(a.p. projection)

# Thorax and Neck

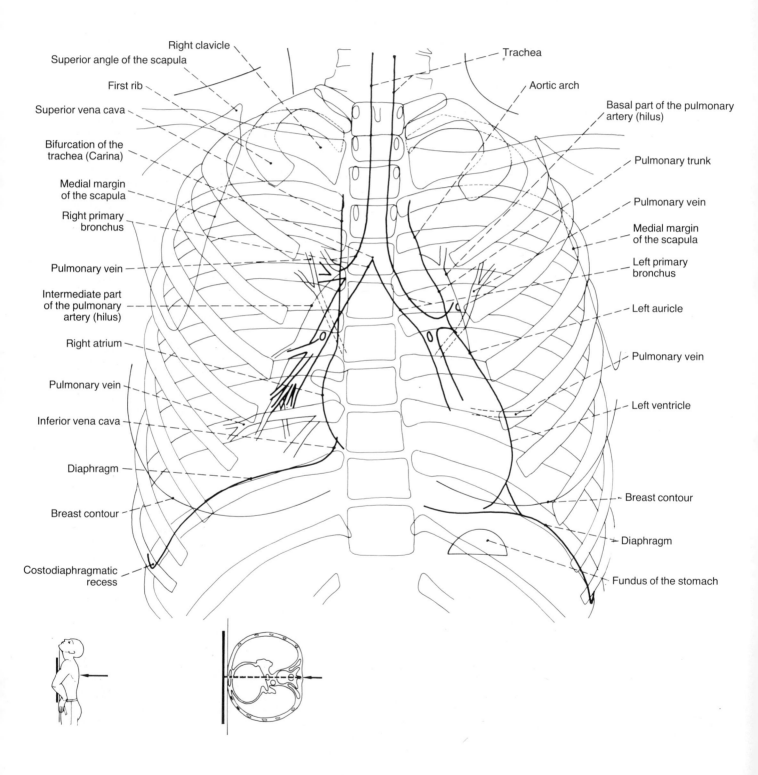

Right clavicle

Trachea

Superior angle of the scapula

Aortic arch

First rib

Basal part of the pulmonary artery (hilus)

Superior vena cava

Pulmonary trunk

Bifurcation of the trachea (Carina)

Pulmonary vein

Medial margin of the scapula

Medial margin of the scapula

Right primary bronchus

Left primary bronchus

Pulmonary vein

Left auricle

Intermediate part of the pulmonary artery (hilus)

Right atrium

Pulmonary vein

Pulmonary vein

Left ventricle

Inferior vena cava

Diaphragm

Breast contour

Breast contour

Diaphragm

Costodiaphragmatic recess

Fundus of the stomach

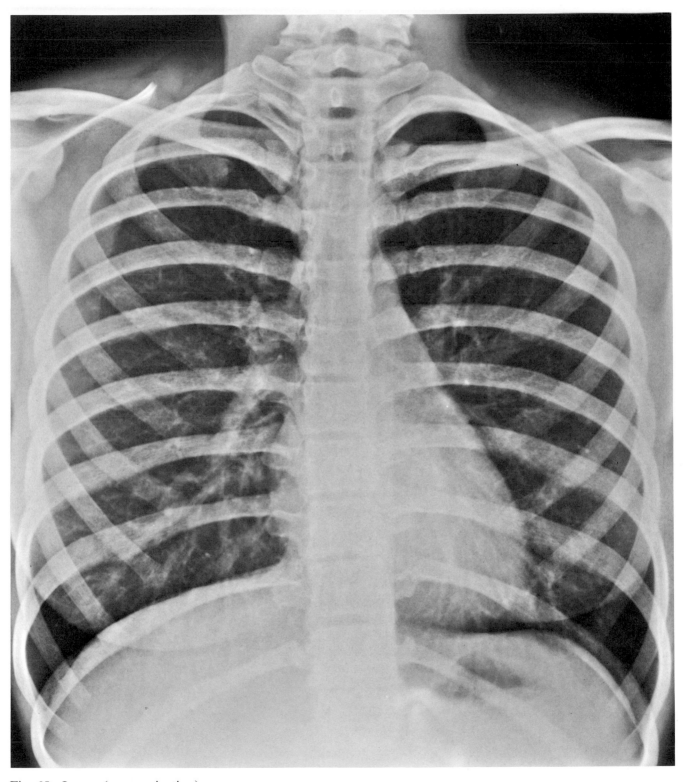

Fig. 69. Lungs (p.a. projection)

# Lungs

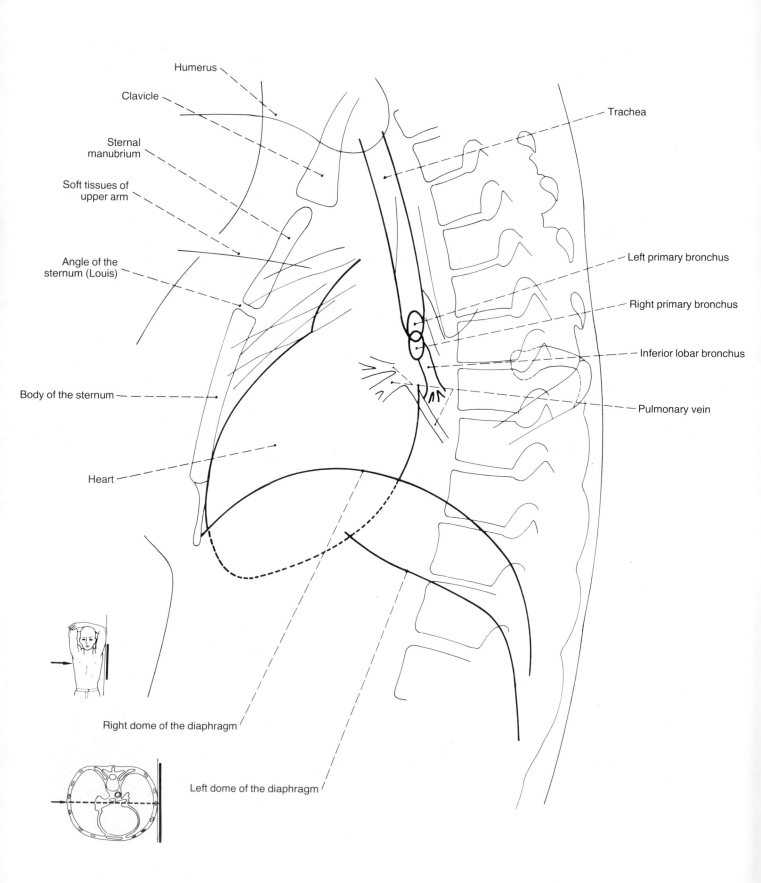

Humerus

Clavicle

Sternal manubrium

Soft tissues of upper arm

Angle of the sternum (Louis)

Body of the sternum

Heart

Trachea

Left primary bronchus

Right primary bronchus

Inferior lobar bronchus

Pulmonary vein

Right dome of the diaphragm

Left dome of the diaphragm

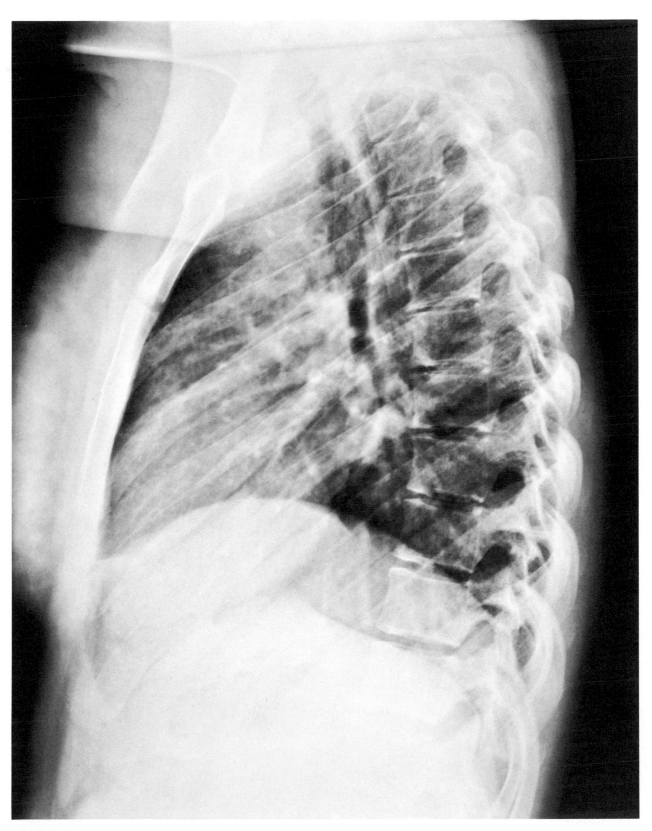

Fig. 70. Lungs (lateral projection)

# Lungs

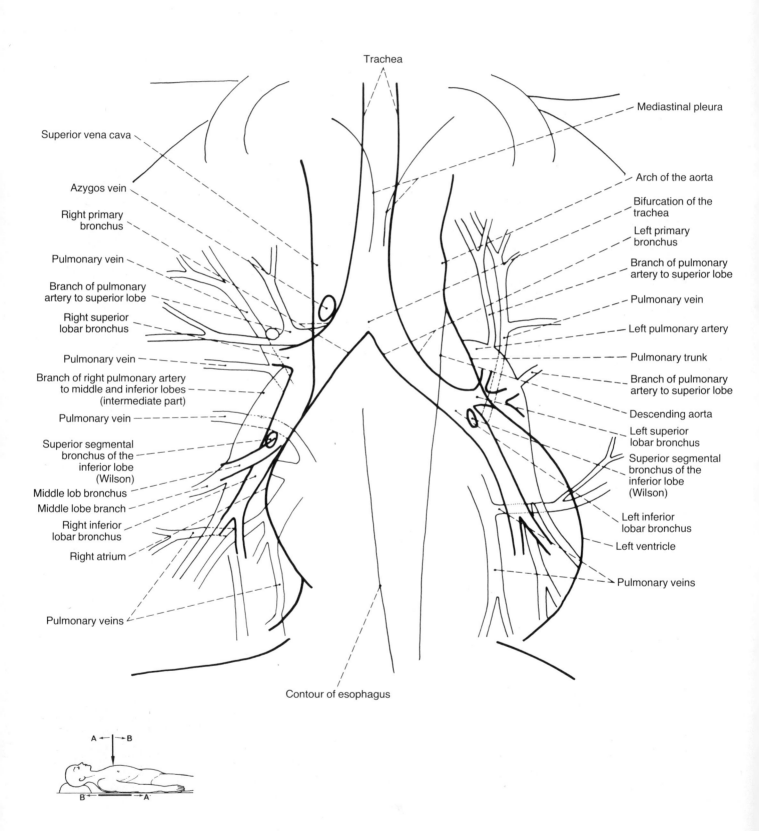

Trachea

Mediastinal pleura

Superior vena cava

Arch of the aorta

Azygos vein

Bifurcation of the trachea

Right primary bronchus

Left primary bronchus

Pulmonary vein

Branch of pulmonary artery to superior lobe

Branch of pulmonary artery to superior lobe

Pulmonary vein

Right superior lobar bronchus

Left pulmonary artery

Pulmonary vein

Pulmonary trunk

Branch of right pulmonary artery to middle and inferior lobes (intermediate part)

Branch of pulmonary artery to superior lobe

Pulmonary vein

Descending aorta

Left superior lobar bronchus

Superior segmental bronchus of the inferior lobe (Wilson)

Superior segmental bronchus of the inferior lobe (Wilson)

Middle lob bronchus

Middle lobe branch

Left inferior lobar bronchus

Right inferior lobar bronchus

Left ventricle

Right atrium

Pulmonary veins

Pulmonary veins

Contour of esophagus

A ← | → B

B ← → A'

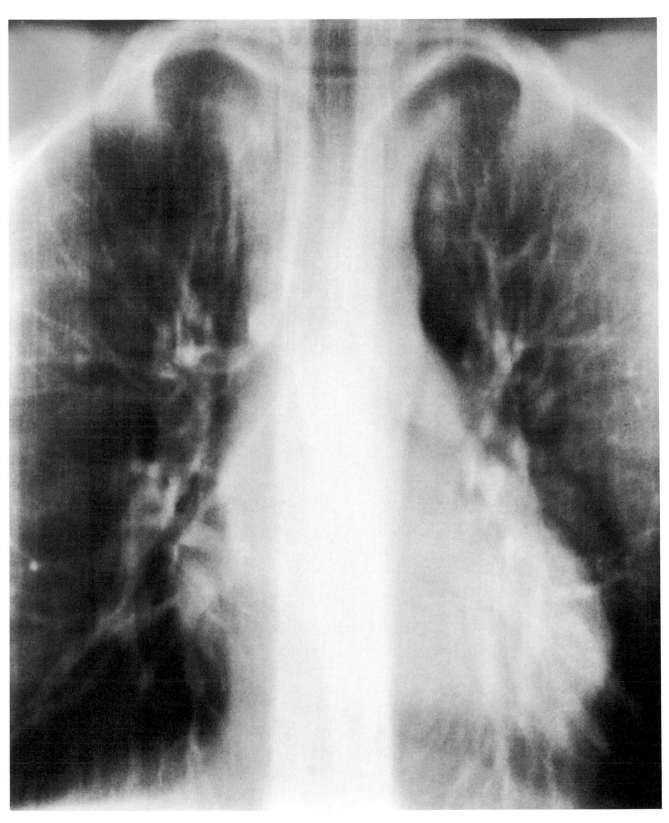

Fig. 71. Tomogram of lungs (a.p. projection)

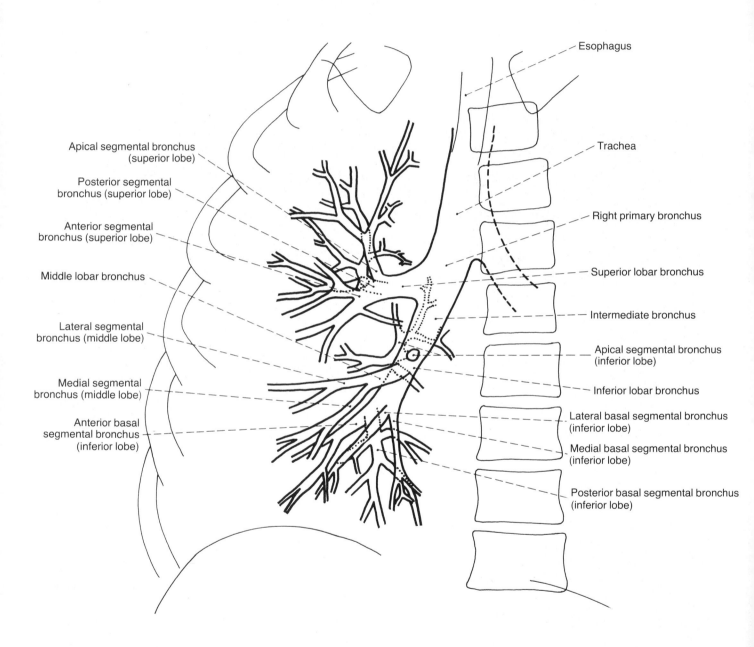

Apical segmental bronchus (superior lobe)

Posterior segmental bronchus (superior lobe)

Anterior segmental bronchus (superior lobe)

Middle lobar bronchus

Lateral segmental bronchus (middle lobe)

Medial segmental bronchus (middle lobe)

Anterior basal segmental bronchus (inferior lobe)

Esophagus

Trachea

Right primary bronchus

Superior lobar bronchus

Intermediate bronchus

Apical segmental bronchus (inferior lobe)

Inferior lobar bronchus

Lateral basal segmental bronchus (inferior lobe)

Medial basal segmental bronchus (inferior lobe)

Posterior basal segmental bronchus (inferior lobe)

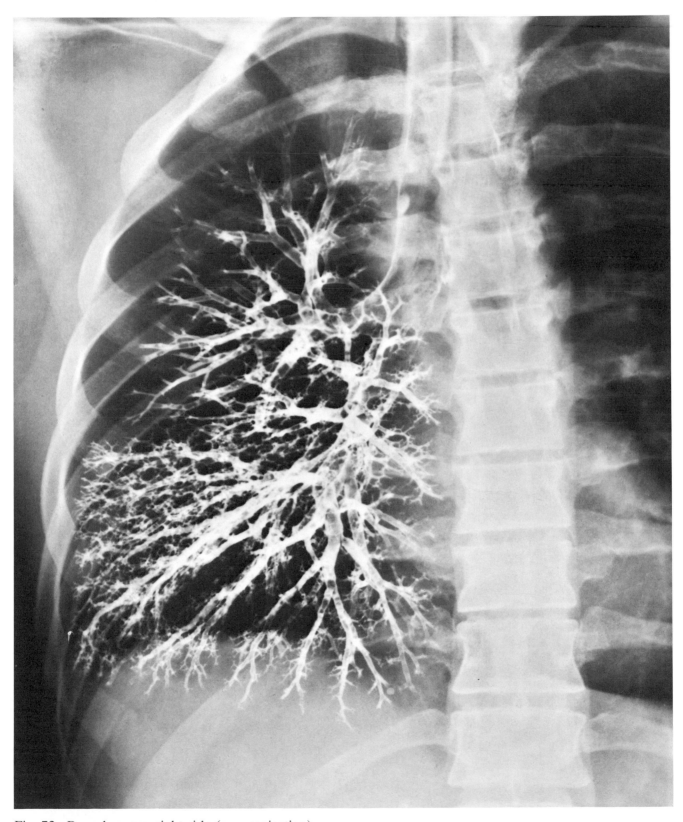

Fig. 72. Bronchogram, right side (a.p. projection)

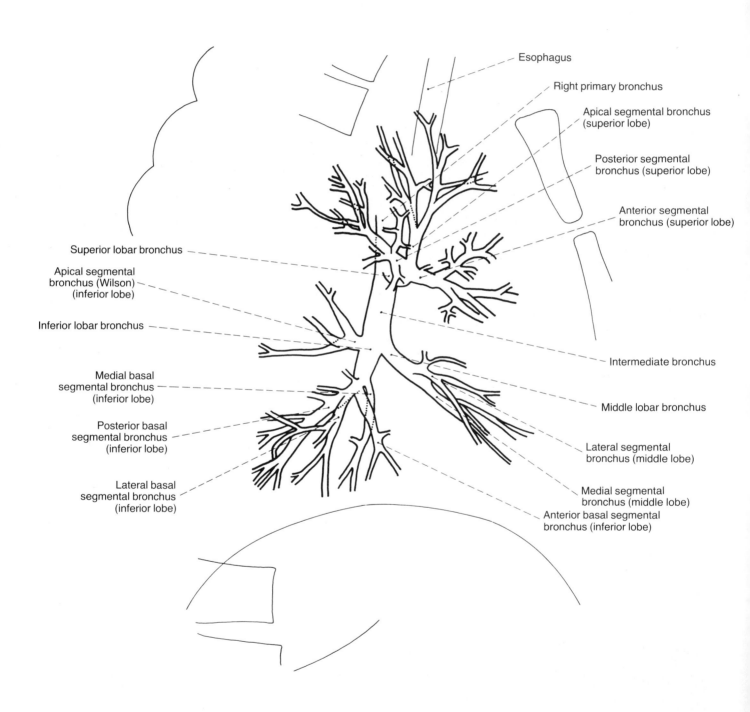

Esophagus

Right primary bronchus

Apical segmental bronchus (superior lobe)

Posterior segmental bronchus (superior lobe)

Anterior segmental bronchus (superior lobe)

Superior lobar bronchus

Apical segmental bronchus (Wilson) (inferior lobe)

Inferior lobar bronchus

Intermediate bronchus

Medial basal segmental bronchus (inferior lobe)

Middle lobar bronchus

Posterior basal segmental bronchus (inferior lobe)

Lateral segmental bronchus (middle lobe)

Lateral basal segmental bronchus (inferior lobe)

Medial segmental bronchus (middle lobe)

Anterior basal segmental bronchus (inferior lobe)

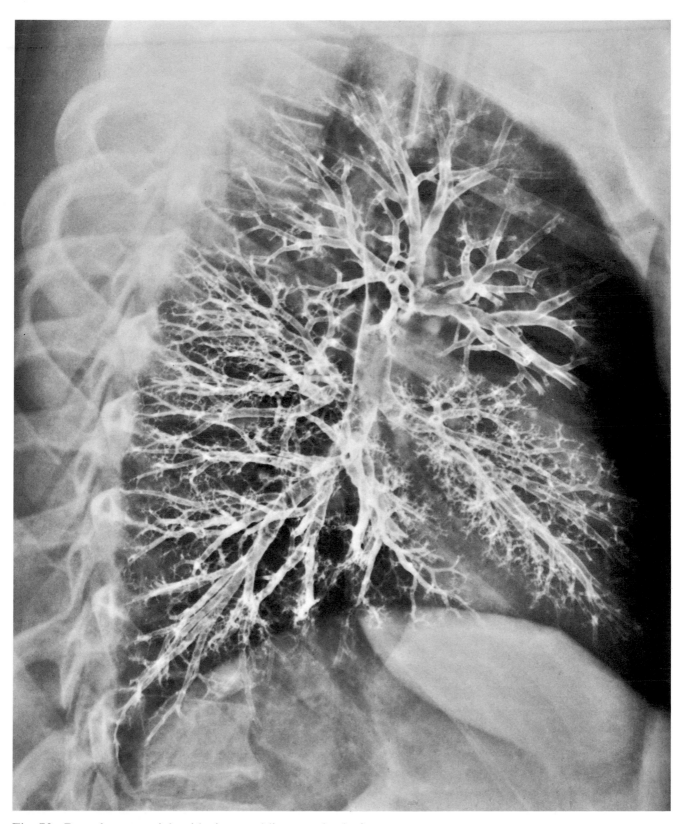

Fig. 73. Bronchogram, right side (steep oblique projection)

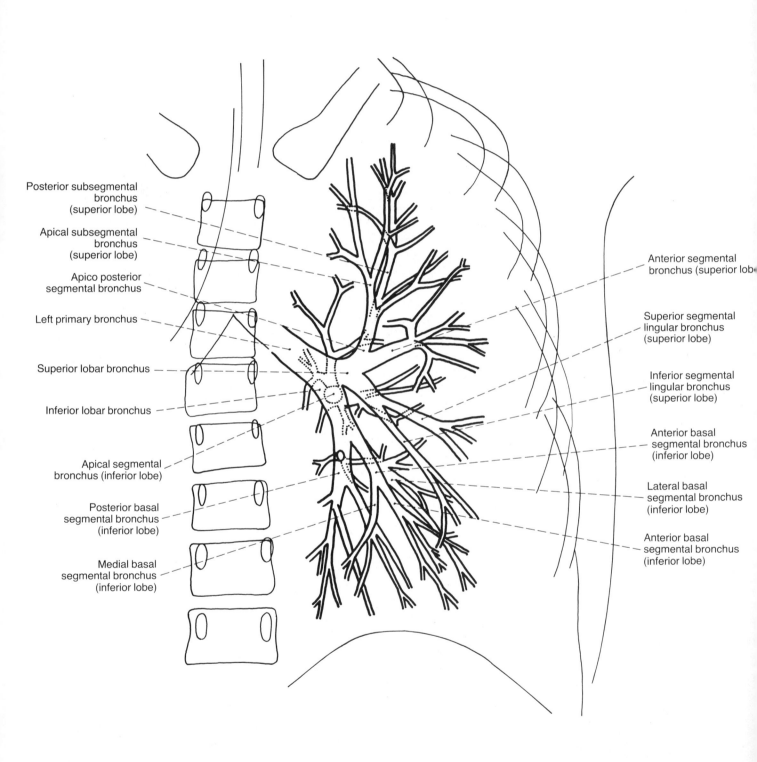

Posterior subsegmental
bronchus
(superior lobe)

Apical subsegmental
bronchus
(superior lobe)

Apico posterior
segmental bronchus

Left primary bronchus

Superior lobar bronchus

Inferior lobar bronchus

Apical segmental
bronchus (inferior lobe)

Posterior basal
segmental bronchus
(inferior lobe)

Medial basal
segmental bronchus
(inferior lobe)

Anterior segmental
bronchus (superior lob

Superior segmental
lingular bronchus
(superior lobe)

Inferior segmental
lingular bronchus
(superior lobe)

Anterior basal
segmental bronchus
(inferior lobe)

Lateral basal
segmental bronchus
(inferior lobe)

Anterior basal
segmental bronchus
(inferior lobe)

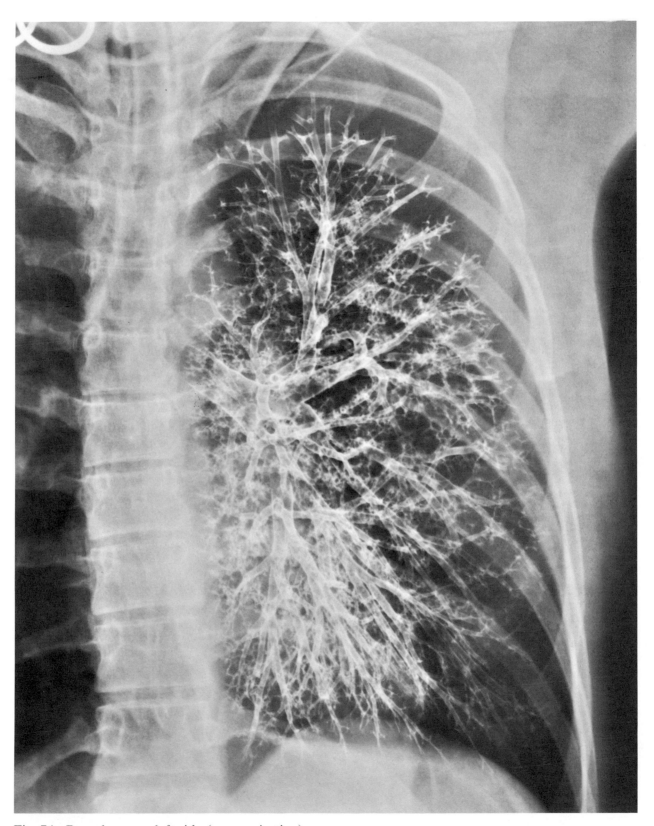

Fig. 74. Bronchogram, left side (a.p. projection)

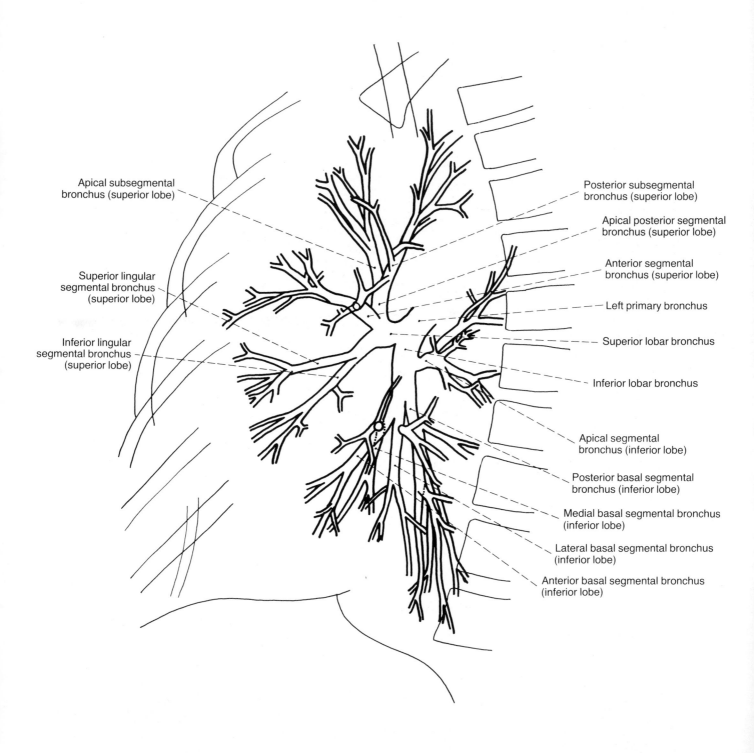

Apical subsegmental
bronchus (superior lobe)

Superior lingular
segmental bronchus
(superior lobe)

Inferior lingular
segmental bronchus
(superior lobe)

Posterior subsegmental
bronchus (superior lobe)

Apical posterior segmental
bronchus (superior lobe)

Anterior segmental
bronchus (superior lobe)

Left primary bronchus

Superior lobar bronchus

Inferior lobar bronchus

Apical segmental
bronchus (inferior lobe)

Posterior basal segmental
bronchus (inferior lobe)

Medial basal segmental bronchus
(inferior lobe)

Lateral basal segmental bronchus
(inferior lobe)

Anterior basal segmental bronchus
(inferior lobe)

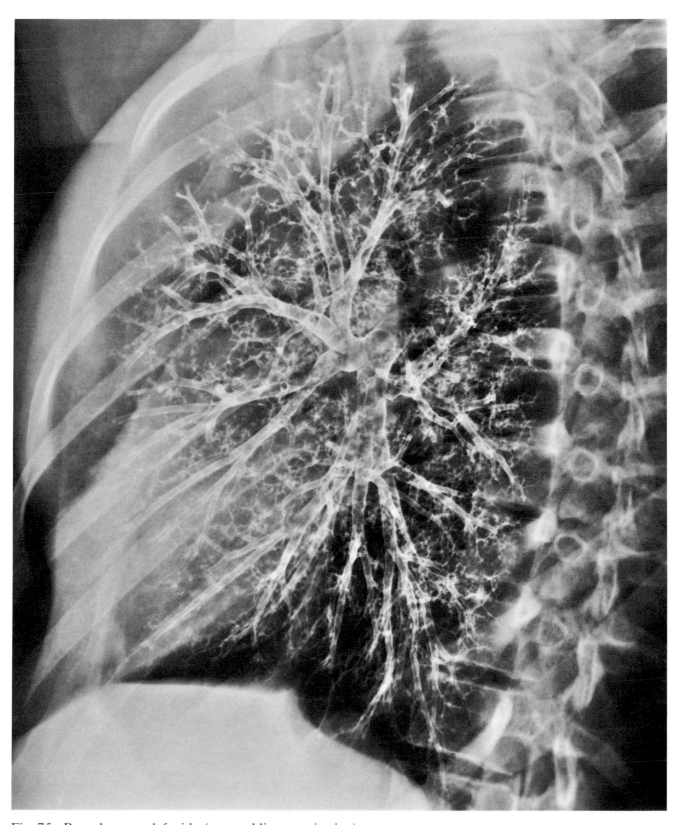

Fig. 75. Bronchogram, left side (steep oblique projection)

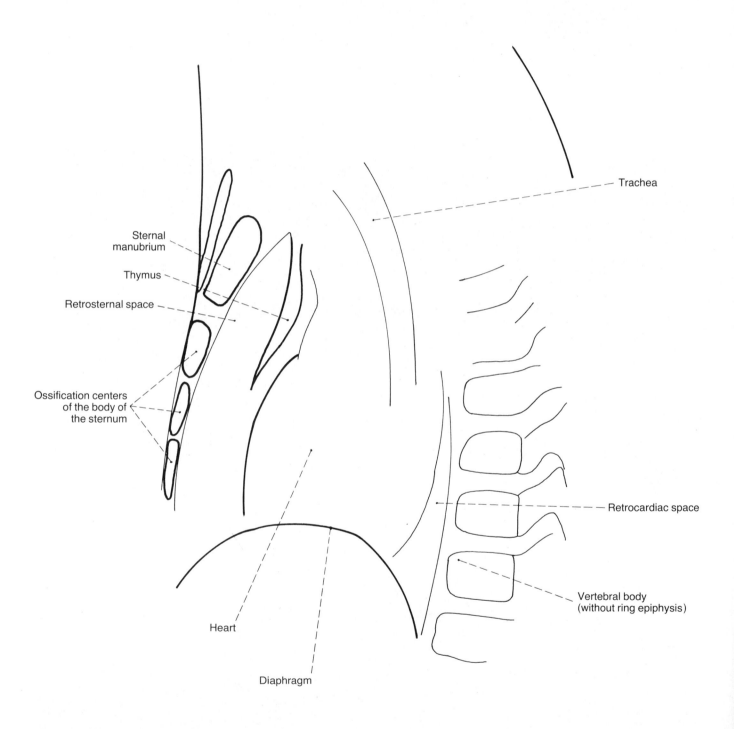

Trachea

Sternal
manubrium

Thymus

Retrosternal space

Ossification centers
of the body of
the sternum

Retrocardiac space

Vertebral body
(without ring epiphysis)

Heart

Diaphragm

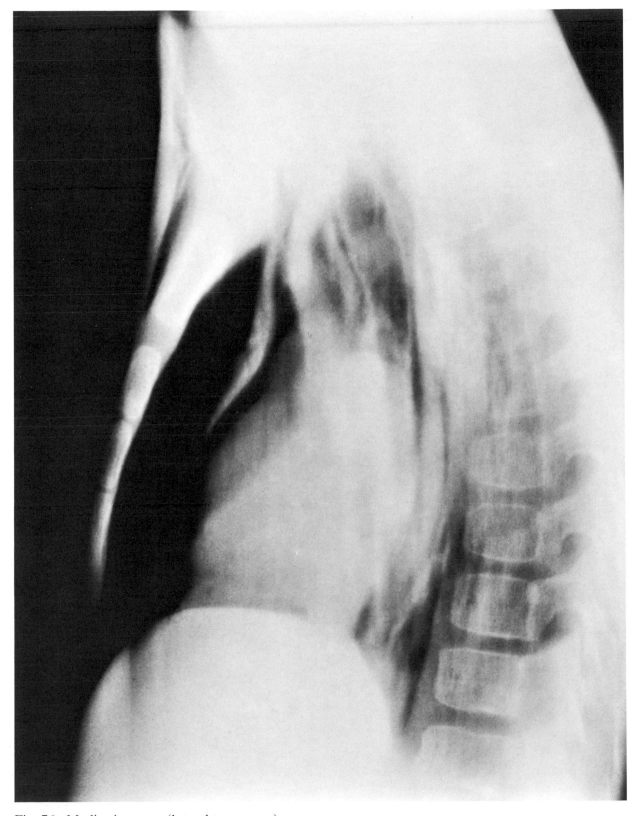

Fig. 76. Mediastinogram (lateral tomogram)

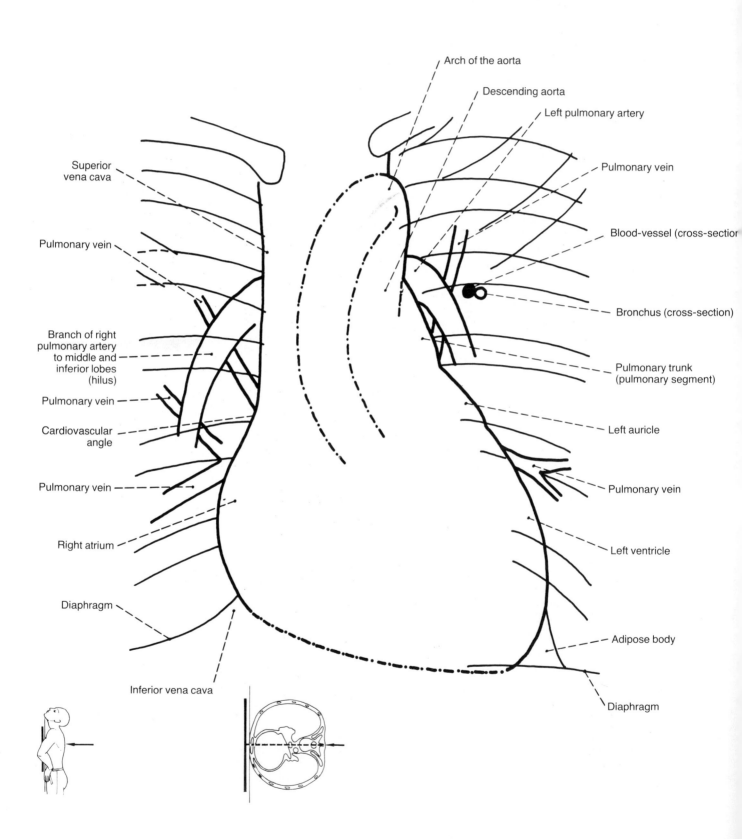

Arch of the aorta

Descending aorta

Left pulmonary artery

Superior vena cava

Pulmonary vein

Pulmonary vein

Blood-vessel (cross-section)

Bronchus (cross-section)

Branch of right pulmonary artery to middle and inferior lobes (hilus)

Pulmonary vein

Pulmonary trunk (pulmonary segment)

Cardiovascular angle

Left auricle

Pulmonary vein

Pulmonary vein

Right atrium

Left ventricle

Diaphragm

Adipose body

Inferior vena cava

Diaphragm

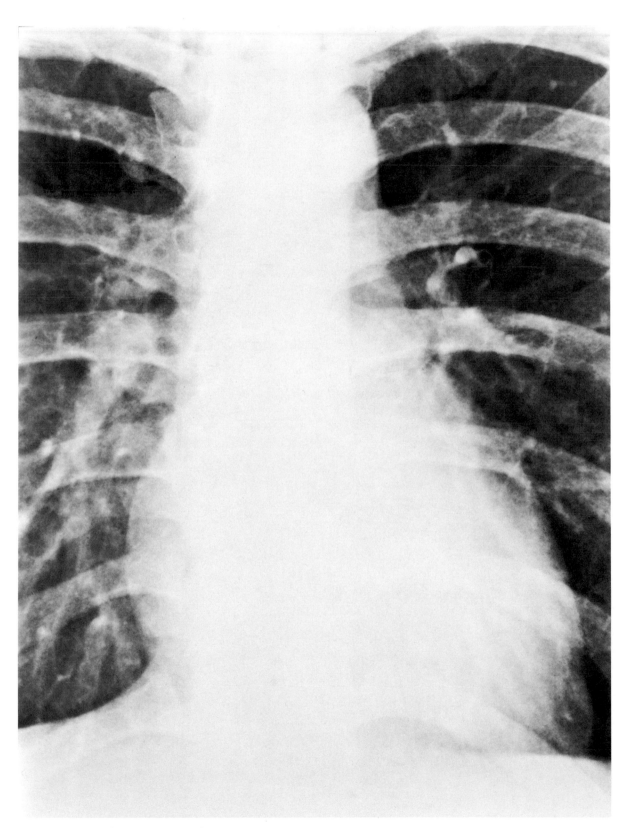

Fig. 77. Heart (p.a. projection)

# Heart

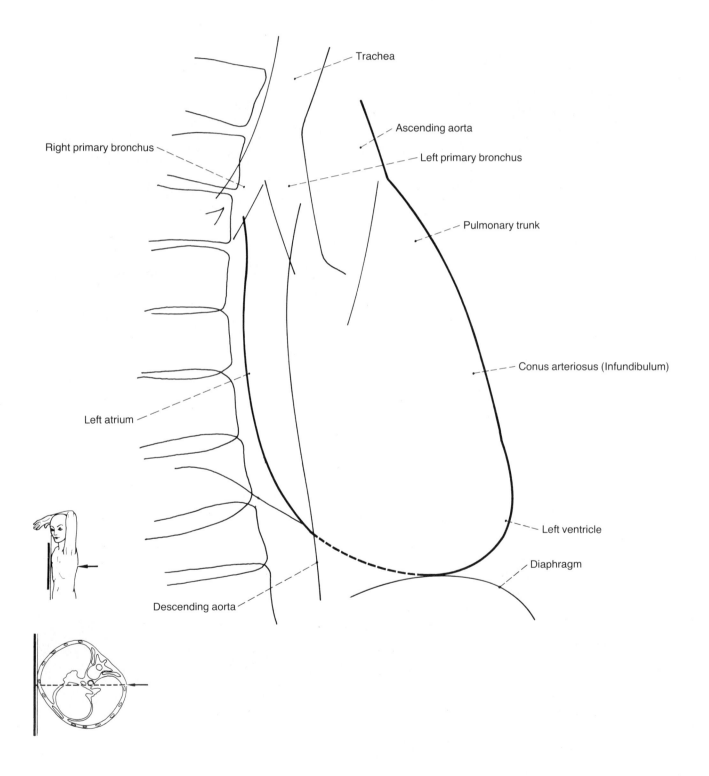

Trachea

Ascending aorta

Right primary bronchus

Left primary bronchus

Pulmonary trunk

Conus arteriosus (Infundibulum)

Left atrium

Left ventricle

Diaphragm

Descending aorta

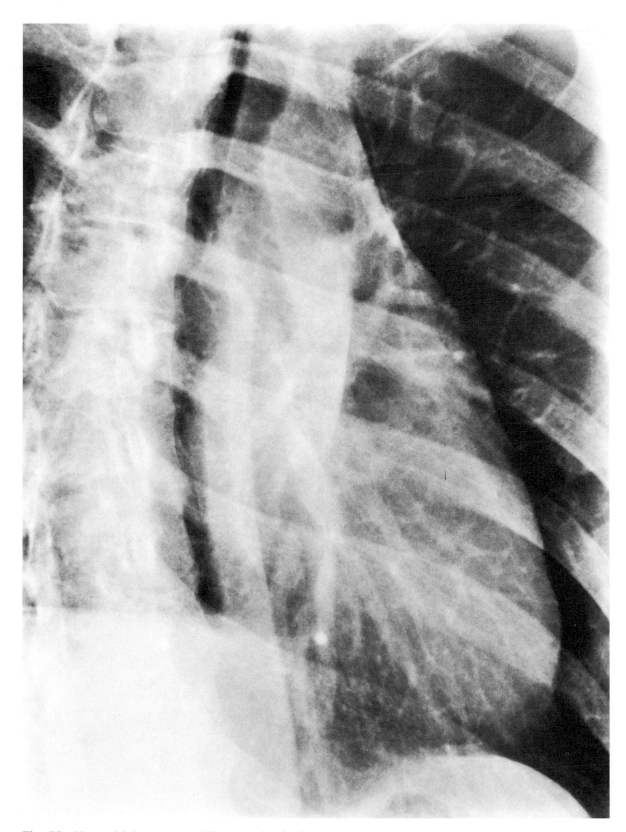

Fig. 78.  Heart (right antero-oblique projection)

# Heart

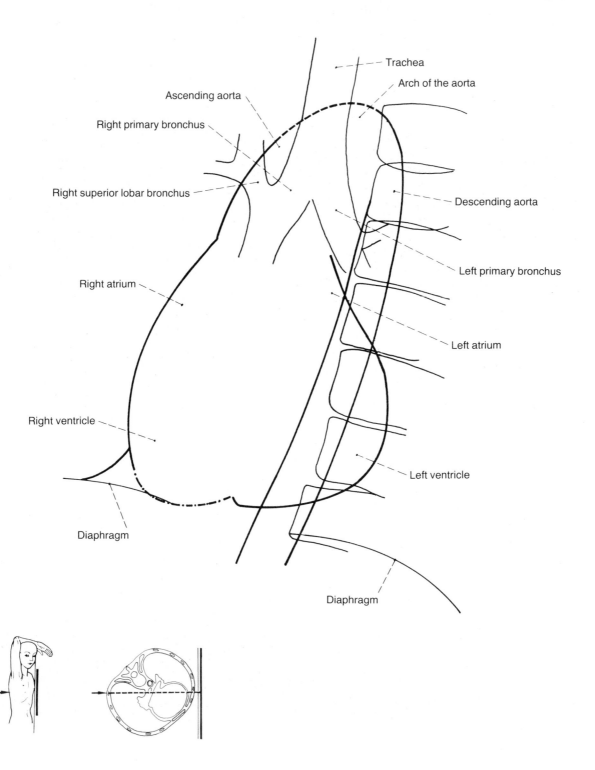

Trachea

Arch of the aorta

Ascending aorta

Right primary bronchus

Right superior lobar bronchus

Descending aorta

Left primary bronchus

Right atrium

Left atrium

Right ventricle

Left ventricle

Diaphragm

Diaphragm

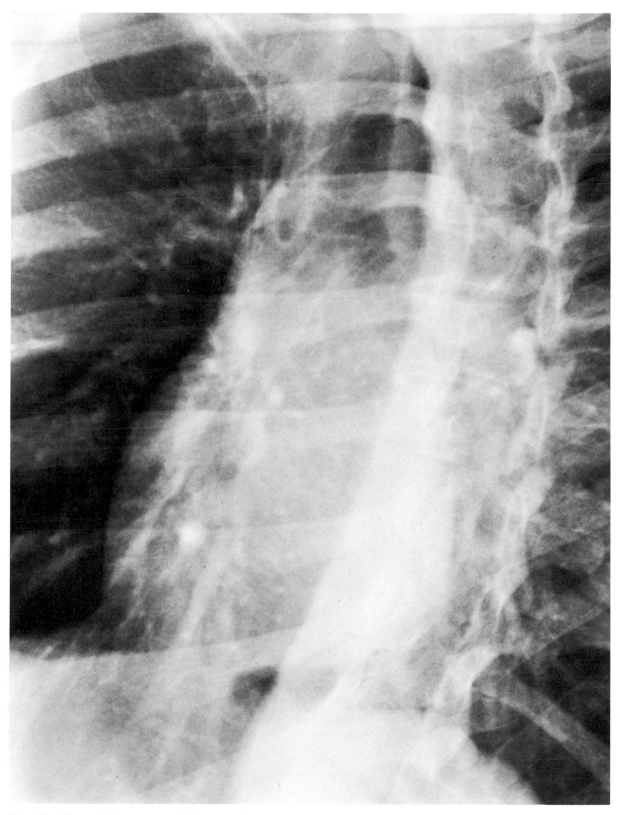

Fig. 79. Heart (left antero-oblique projection)

# Heart

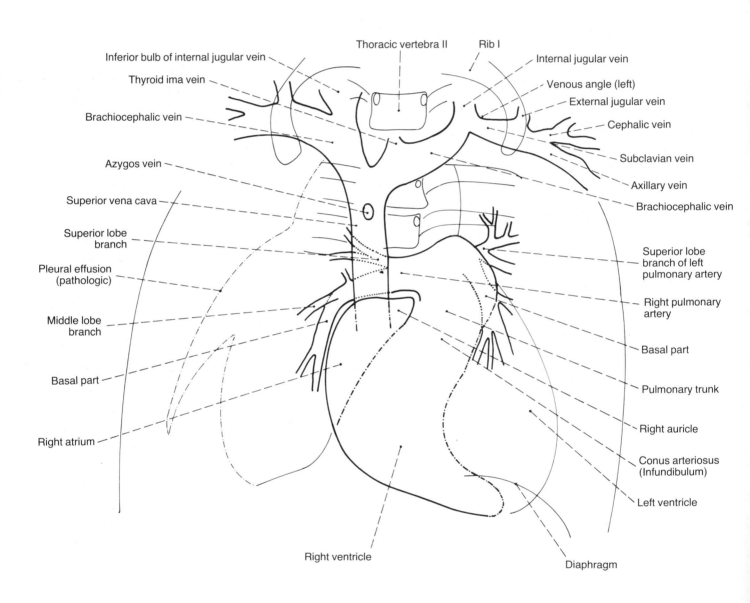

Inferior bulb of internal jugular vein

Thyroid ima vein

Brachiocephalic vein

Azygos vein

Superior vena cava

Superior lobe branch

Pleural effusion (pathologic)

Middle lobe branch

Basal part

Right atrium

Thoracic vertebra II

Rib I

Internal jugular vein

Venous angle (left)

External jugular vein

Cephalic vein

Subclavian vein

Axillary vein

Brachiocephalic vein

Superior lobe branch of left pulmonary artery

Right pulmonary artery

Basal part

Pulmonary trunk

Right auricle

Conus arteriosus (Infundibulum)

Left ventricle

Right ventricle

Diaphragm

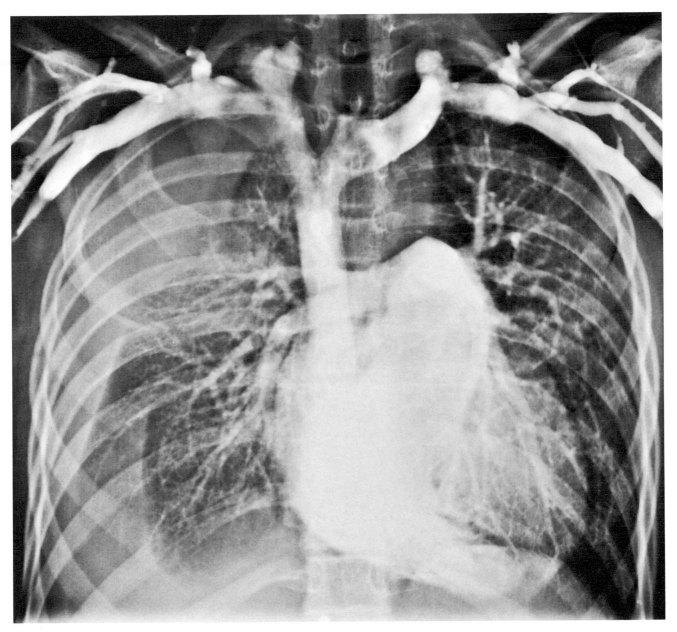

Fig. 80. Venous angiocardiography

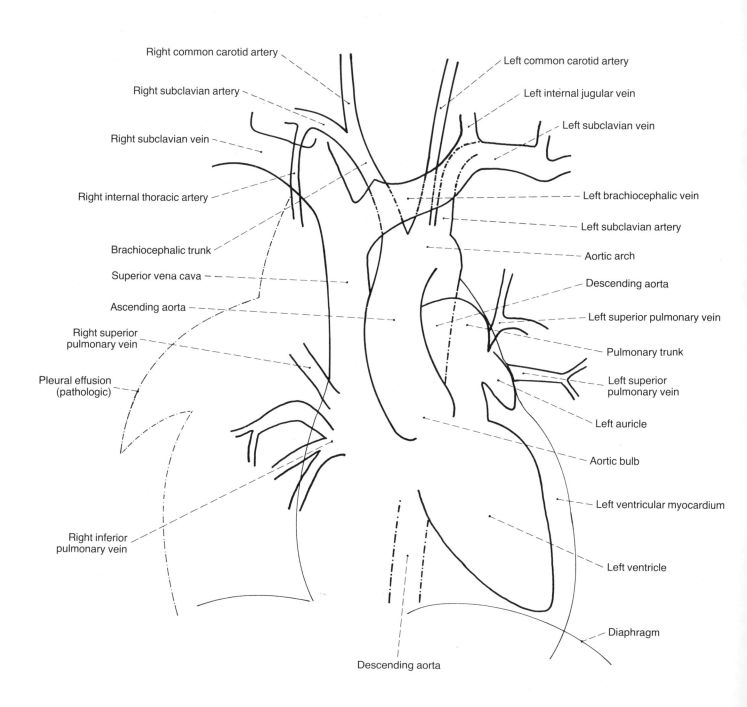

Right common carotid artery

Right subclavian artery

Right subclavian vein

Right internal thoracic artery

Brachiocephalic trunk

Superior vena cava

Ascending aorta

Right superior
pulmonary vein

Pleural effusion
(pathologic)

Right inferior
pulmonary vein

Left common carotid artery

Left internal jugular vein

Left subclavian vein

Left brachiocephalic vein

Left subclavian artery

Aortic arch

Descending aorta

Left superior pulmonary vein

Pulmonary trunk

Left superior
pulmonary vein

Left auricle

Aortic bulb

Left ventricular myocardium

Left ventricle

Diaphragm

Descending aorta

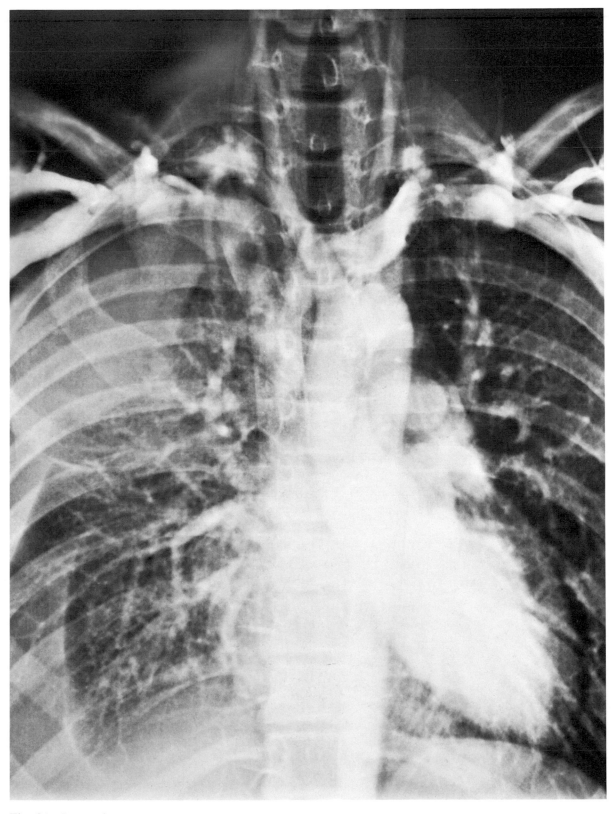

Fig. 81. Levo phase

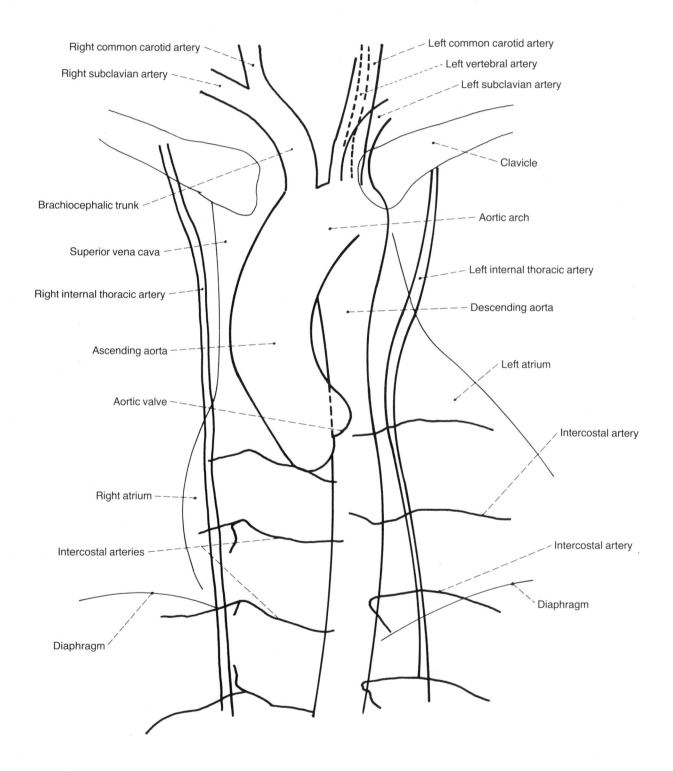

Right common carotid artery

Right subclavian artery

Left common carotid artery

Left vertebral artery

Left subclavian artery

Clavicle

Brachiocephalic trunk

Aortic arch

Superior vena cava

Left internal thoracic artery

Right internal thoracic artery

Descending aorta

Ascending aorta

Left atrium

Aortic valve

Intercostal artery

Right atrium

Intercostal arteries

Intercostal artery

Diaphragm

Diaphragm

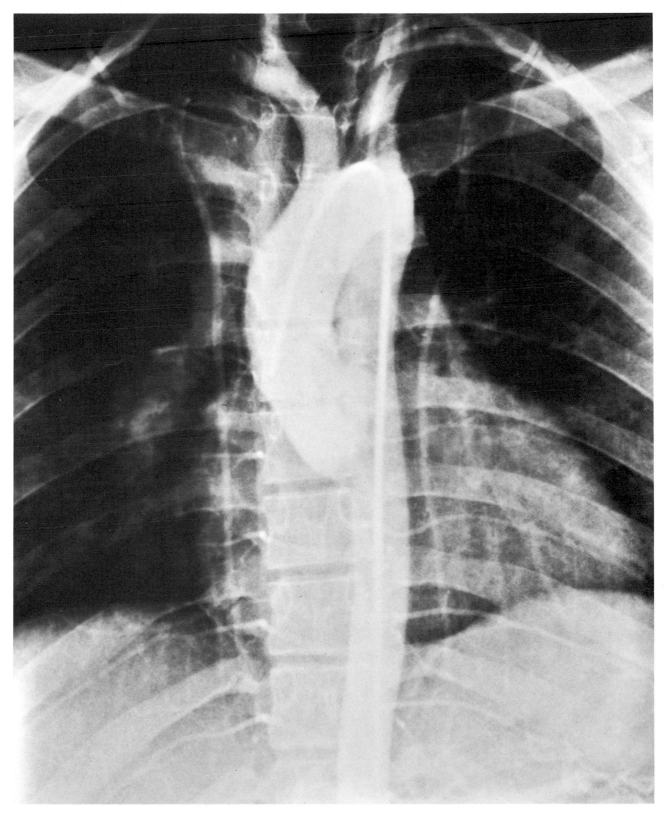

Fig. 82. Aortic arch

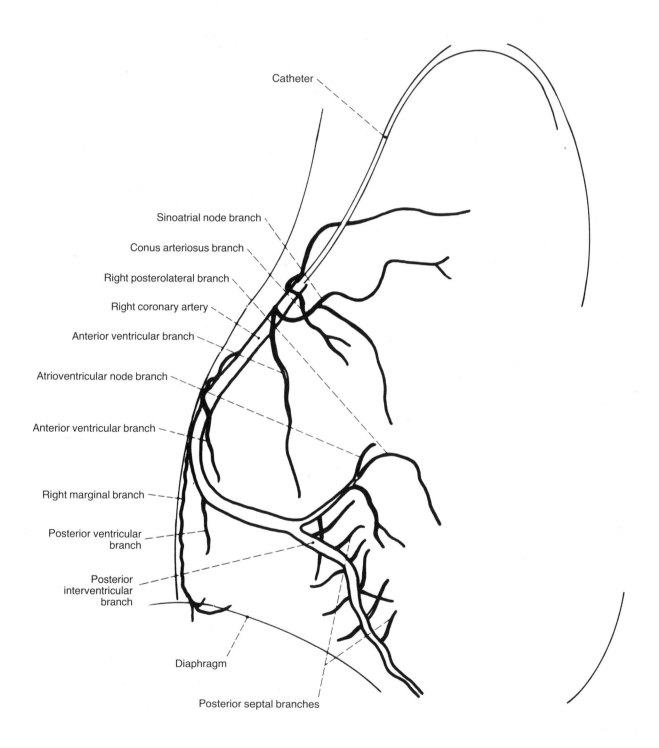

Catheter

Sinoatrial node branch

Conus arteriosus branch

Right posterolateral branch

Right coronary artery

Anterior ventricular branch

Atrioventricular node branch

Anterior ventricular branch

Right marginal branch

Posterior ventricular branch

Posterior interventricular branch

Diaphragm

Posterior septal branches

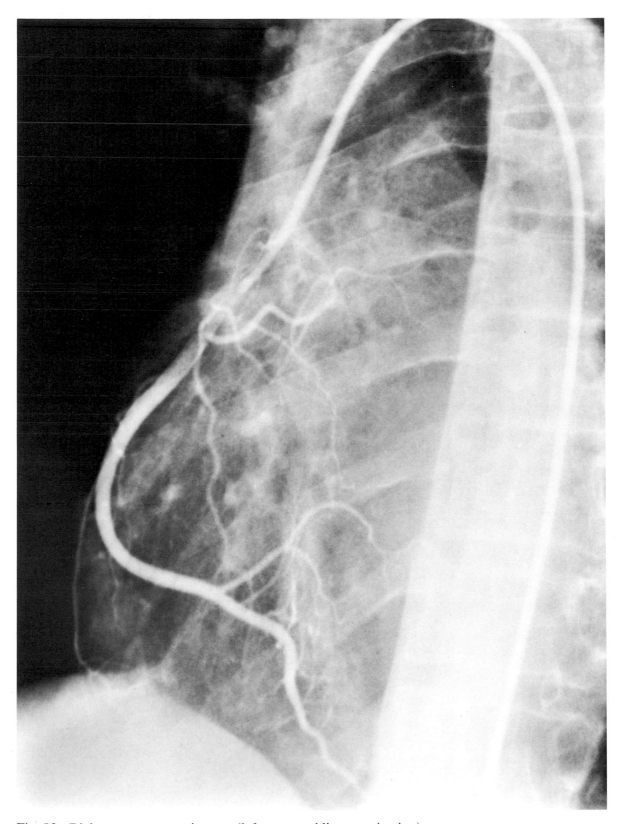

Fig. 83. Right coronary arteriogram (left antero-oblique projection)

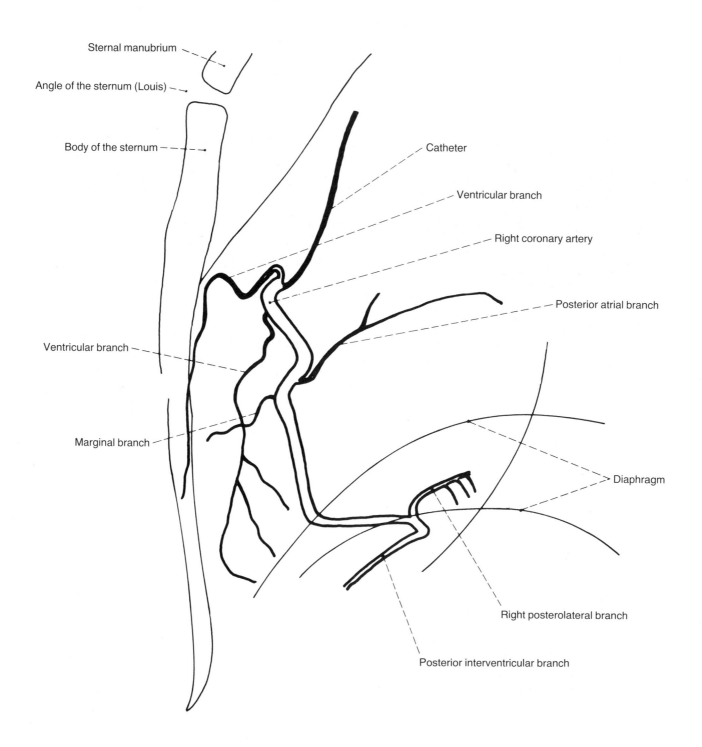

Sternal manubrium

Angle of the sternum (Louis)

Body of the sternum

Catheter

Ventricular branch

Right coronary artery

Posterior atrial branch

Ventricular branch

Marginal branch

Diaphragm

Right posterolateral branch

Posterior interventricular branch

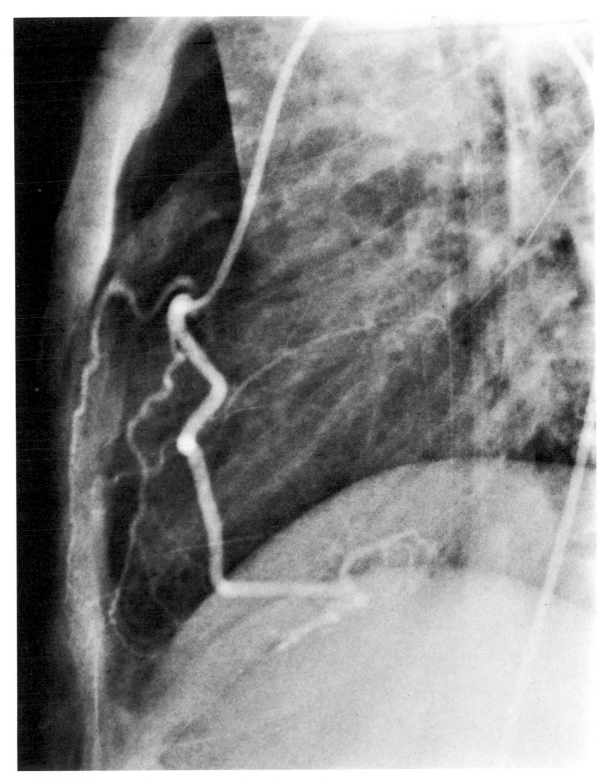

Fig. 84. Right coronary arteriogram (lateral projection)

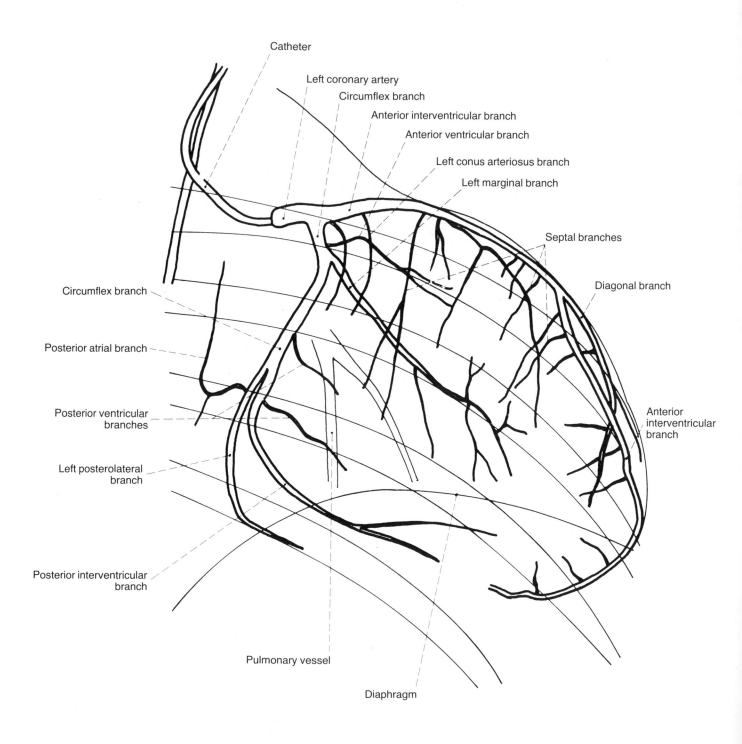

Catheter

Left coronary artery

Circumflex branch

Anterior interventricular branch

Anterior ventricular branch

Left conus arteriosus branch

Left marginal branch

Septal branches

Diagonal branch

Circumflex branch

Posterior atrial branch

Posterior ventricular
branches

Anterior
interventricular
branch

Left posterolateral
branch

Posterior interventricular
branch

Pulmonary vessel

Diaphragm

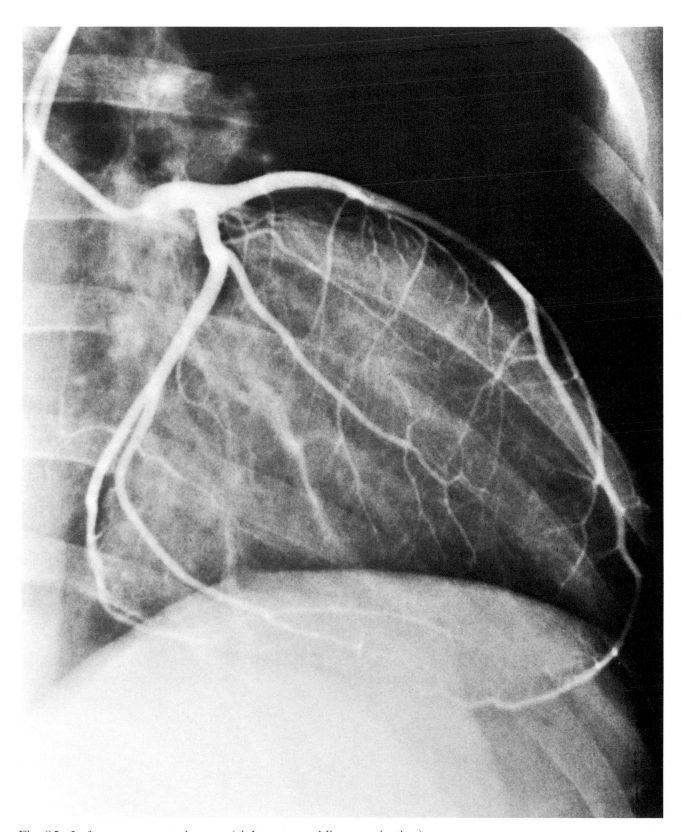

Fig. 85. Left coronary arteriogram (right antero-oblique projection)

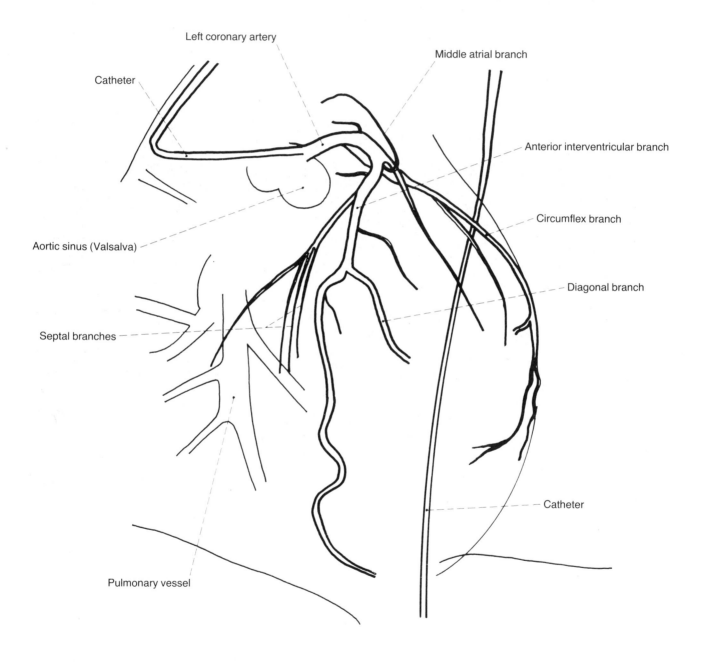

Left coronary artery

Catheter

Middle atrial branch

Anterior interventricular branch

Circumflex branch

Aortic sinus (Valsalva)

Diagonal branch

Septal branches

Catheter

Pulmonary vessel

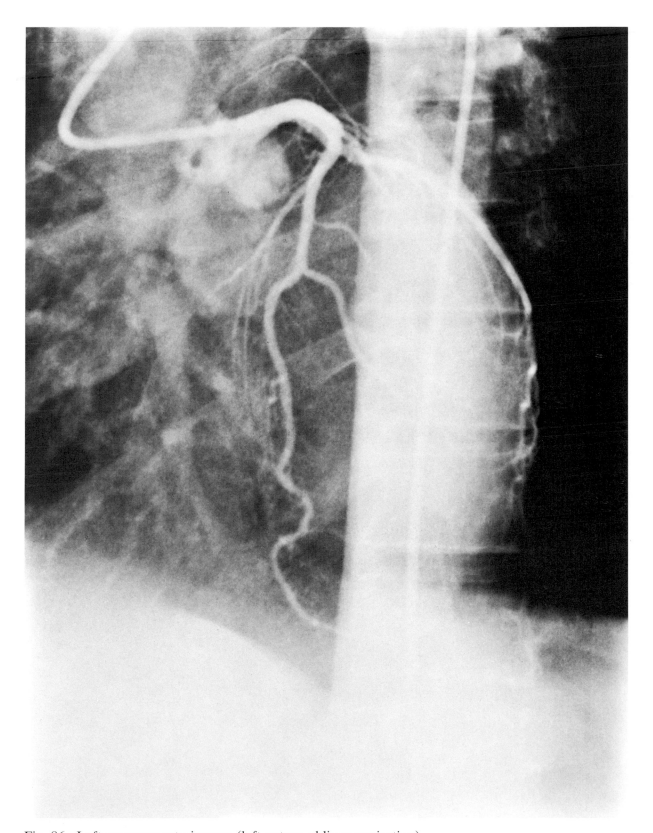

Fig. 86. Left coronary arteriogram (left antero-oblique projection)

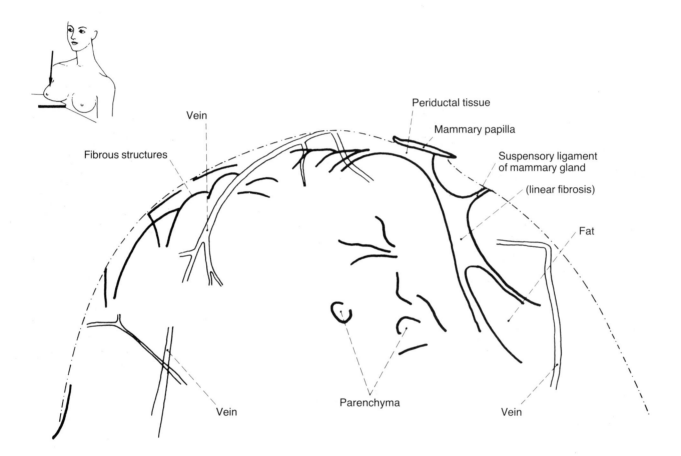

Vein

Periductal tissue

Mammary papilla

Fibrous structures

Suspensory ligament
of mammary gland

(linear fibrosis)

Fat

Vein

Parenchyma

Vein

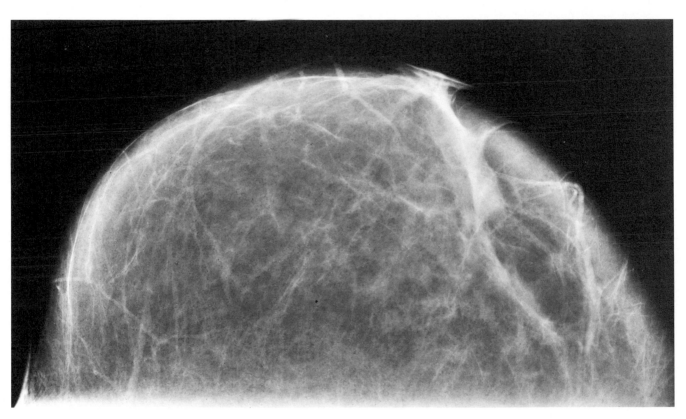

Fig. 87. Mammogram (cranio-caudal projection)

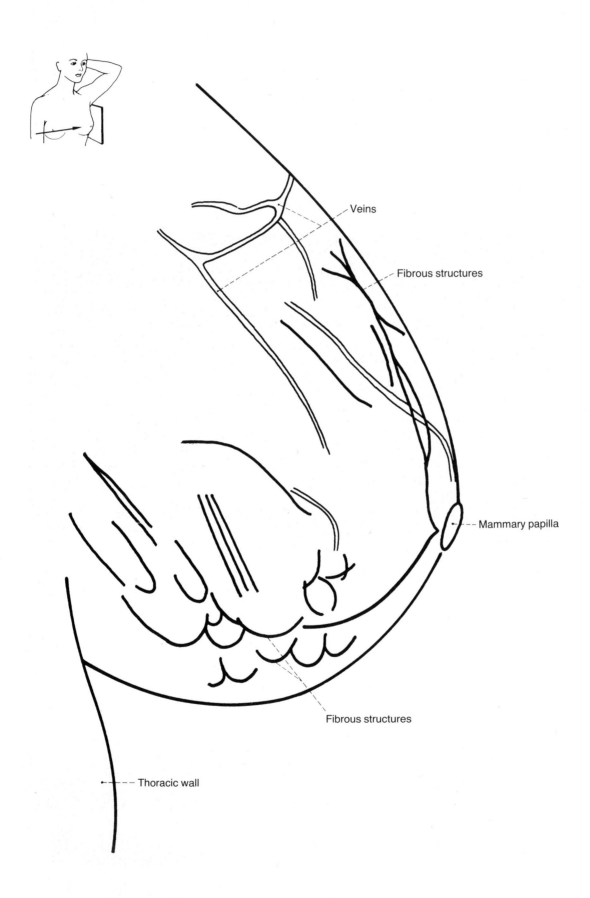

Veins

Fibrous structures

Mammary papilla

Fibrous structures

Thoracic wall

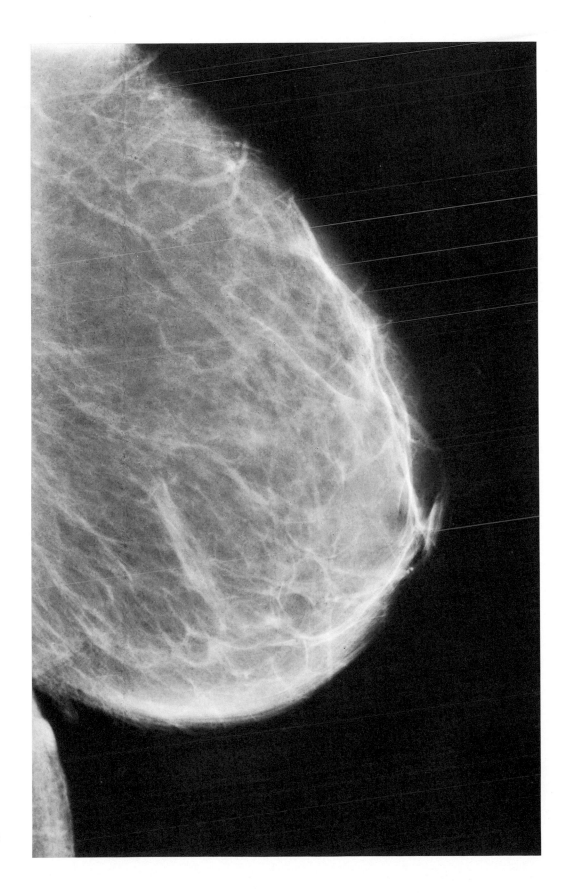

Fig. 88. Mammogram
(lateral projection)

# Trachea

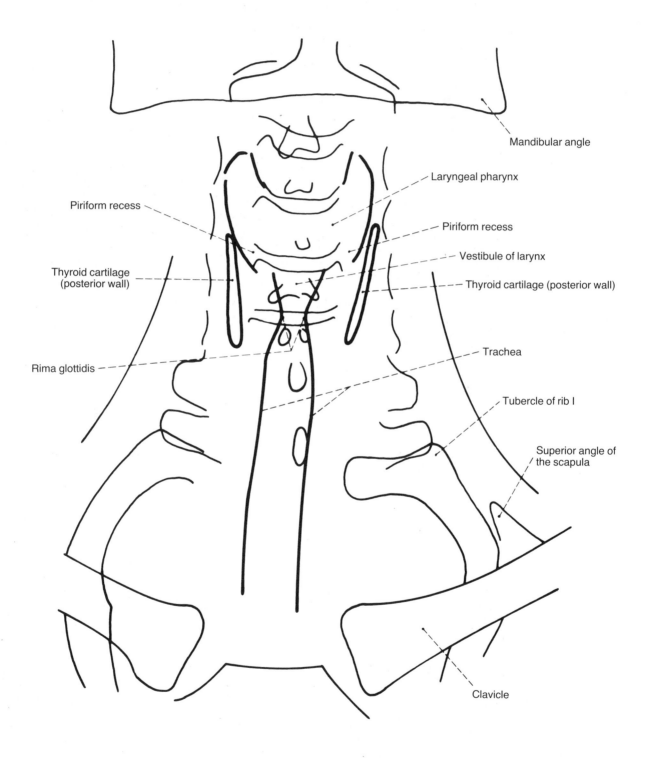

Mandibular angle

Laryngeal pharynx

Piriform recess

Piriform recess

Vestibule of larynx

Thyroid cartilage
(posterior wall)

Thyroid cartilage (posterior wall)

Trachea

Rima glottidis

Tubercle of rib I

Superior angle of
the scapula

Clavicle

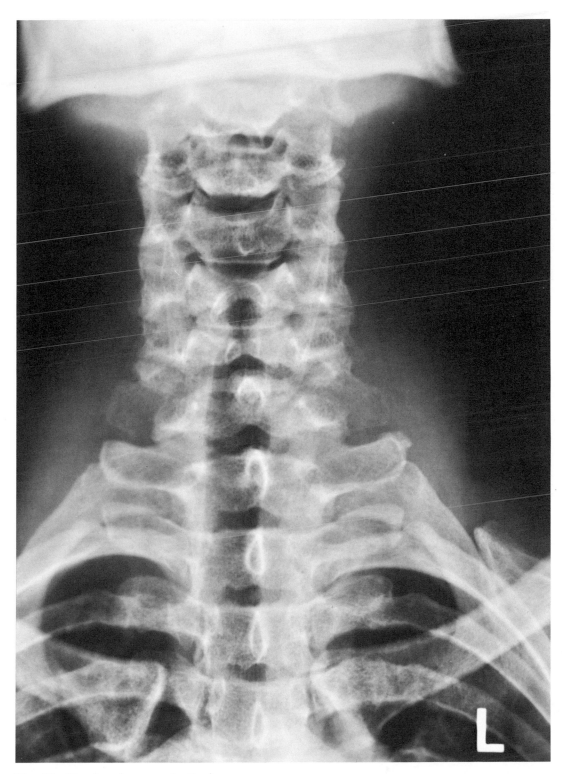

Fig. 89. Trachea (a. p. projection)

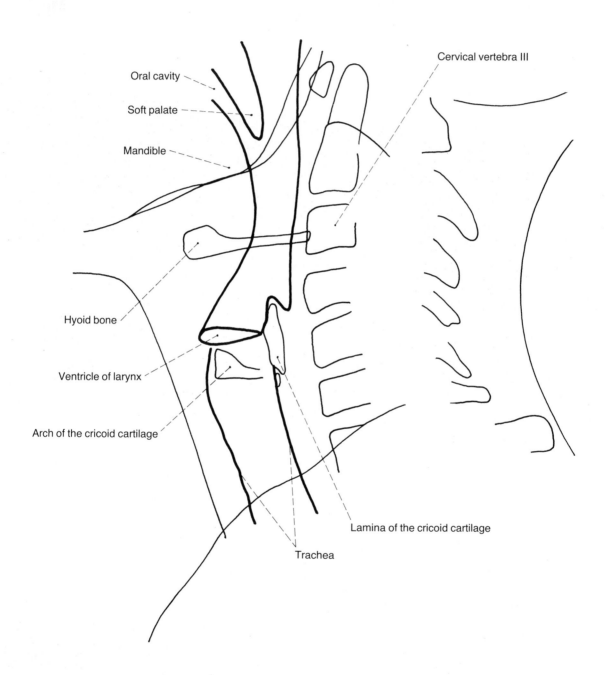

Oral cavity

Soft palate

Mandible

Hyoid bone

Ventricle of larynx

Arch of the cricoid cartilage

Cervical vertebra III

Lamina of the cricoid cartilage

Trachea

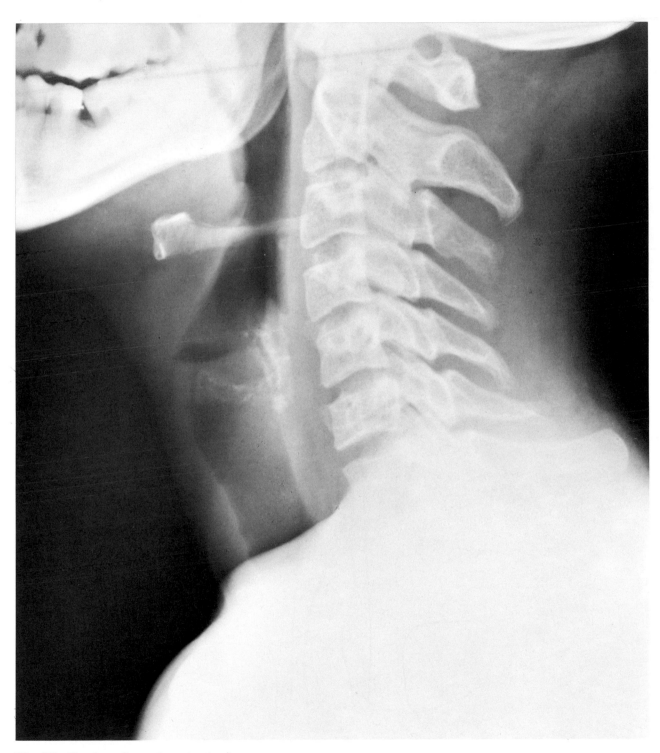

Fig. 90. Trachea (lateral projection)

# Digestive Tract

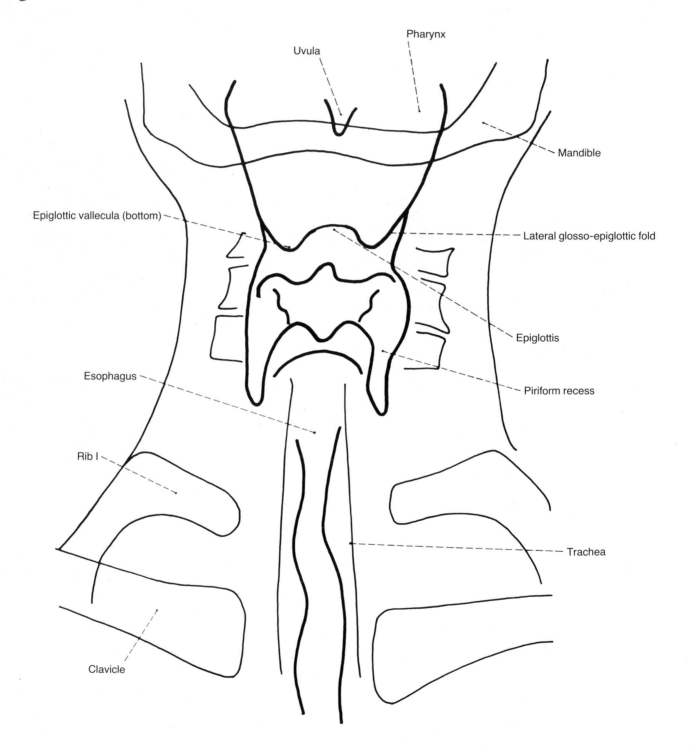

Uvula

Pharynx

Mandible

Epiglottic vallecula (bottom)

Lateral glosso-epiglottic fold

Epiglottis

Esophagus

Piriform recess

Rib I

Trachea

Clavicle

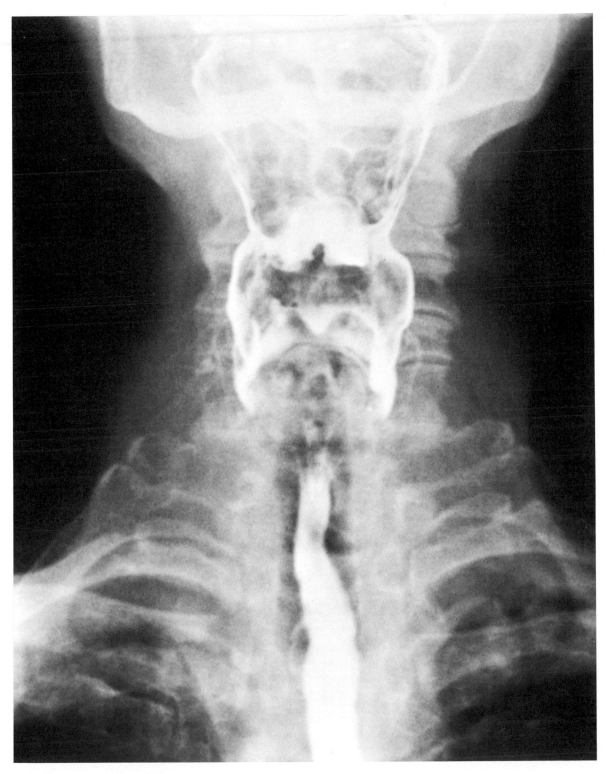

Fig. 91. Act of swallowing (p.a. projection)

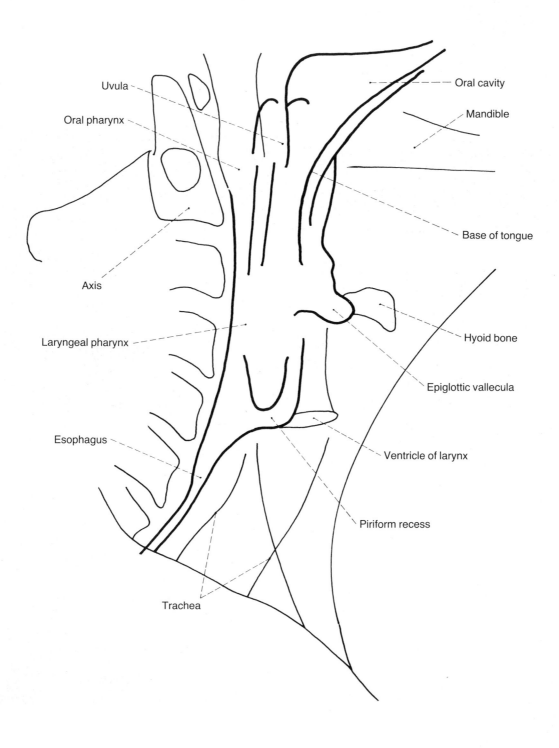

Uvula

Oral pharynx

Axis

Laryngeal pharynx

Esophagus

Trachea

Oral cavity

Mandible

Base of tongue

Hyoid bone

Epiglottic vallecula

Ventricle of larynx

Piriform recess

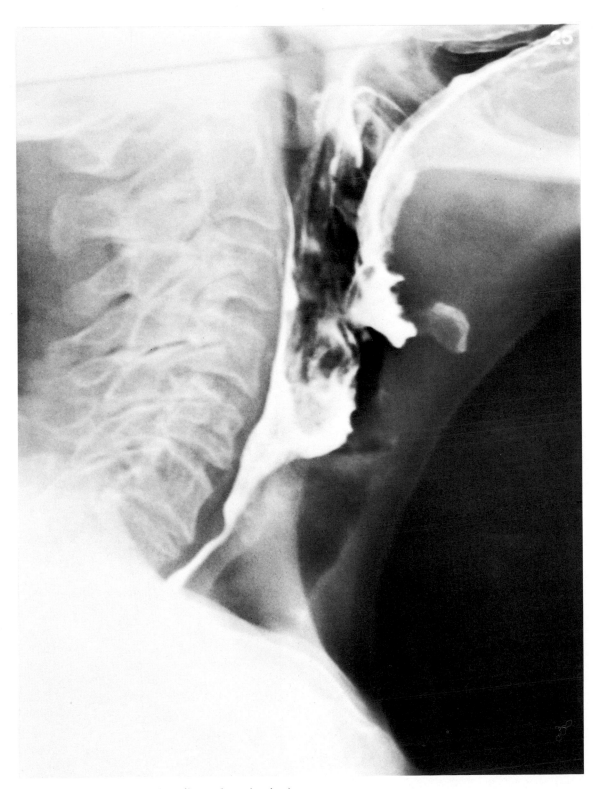

Fig. 92. Act of swallowing (lateral projection)

# Esophagus

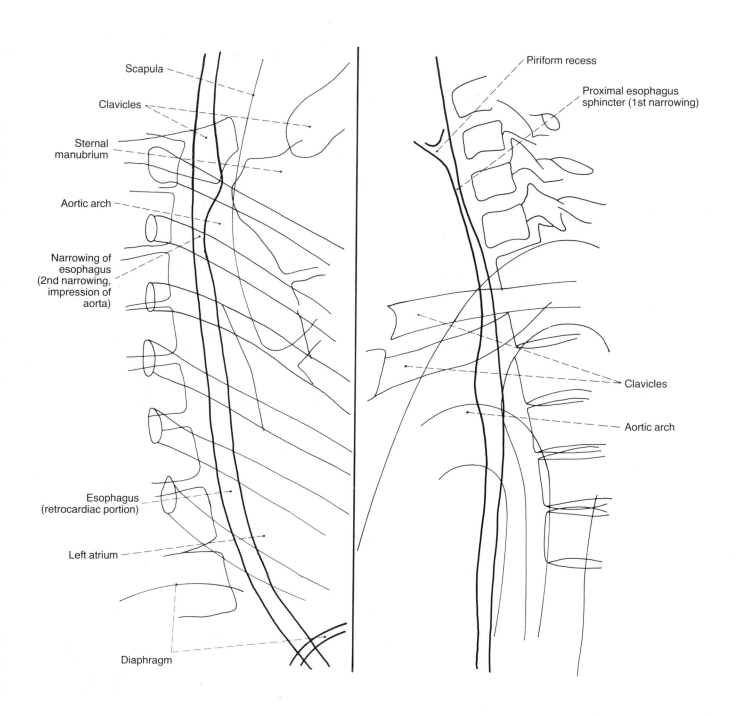

Scapula

Clavicles

Sternal
manubrium

Aortic arch

Narrowing of
esophagus
(2nd narrowing,
impression of
aorta)

Esophagus
(retrocardiac portion)

Left atrium

Diaphragm

Piriform recess

Proximal esophagus
sphincter (1st narrowing)

Clavicles

Aortic arch

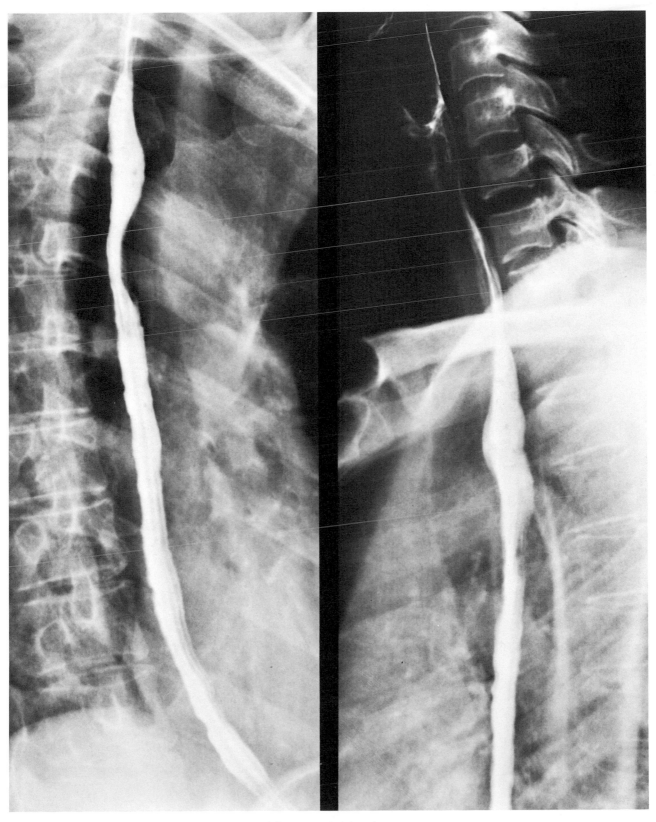

Fig. 93. Esophagus (right and left antero-oblique projections)

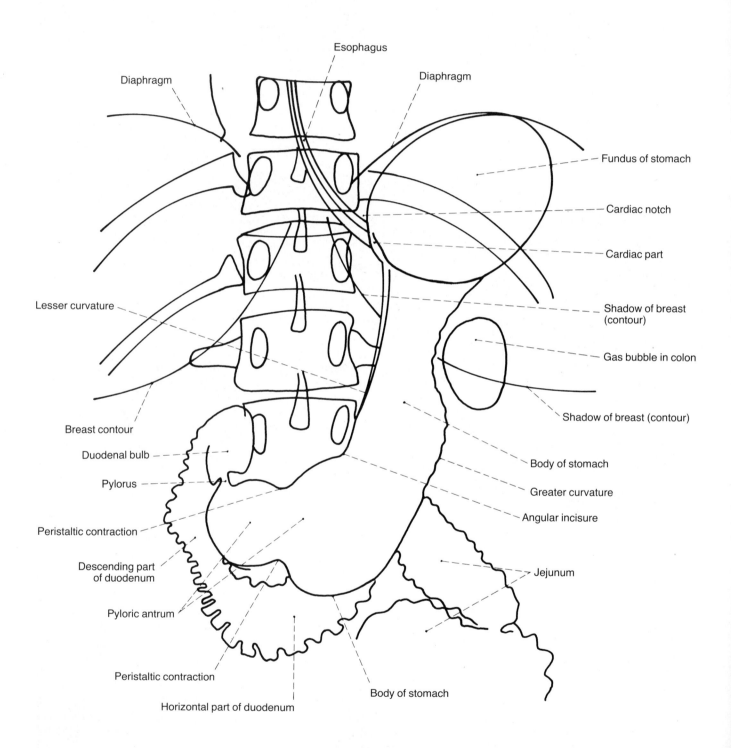

Esophagus

Diaphragm

Diaphragm

Fundus of stomach

Cardiac notch

Cardiac part

Lesser curvature

Shadow of breast (contour)

Gas bubble in colon

Shadow of breast (contour)

Breast contour

Duodenal bulb

Body of stomach

Pylorus

Greater curvature

Angular incisure

Peristaltic contraction

Descending part of duodenum

Jejunum

Pyloric antrum

Peristaltic contraction

Body of stomach

Horizontal part of duodenum

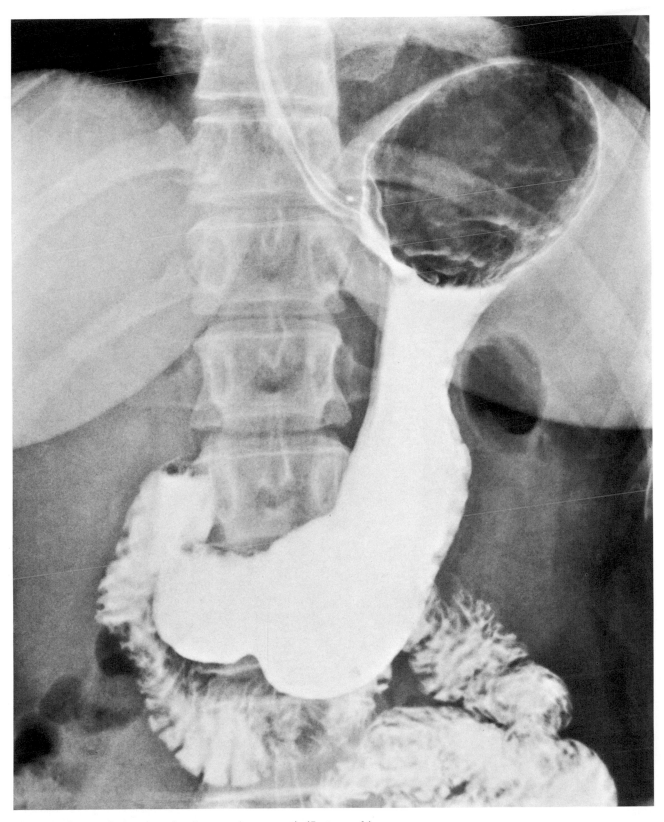

Fig. 94. Stomach (p.a. projection, patient erect) (J-stomach)

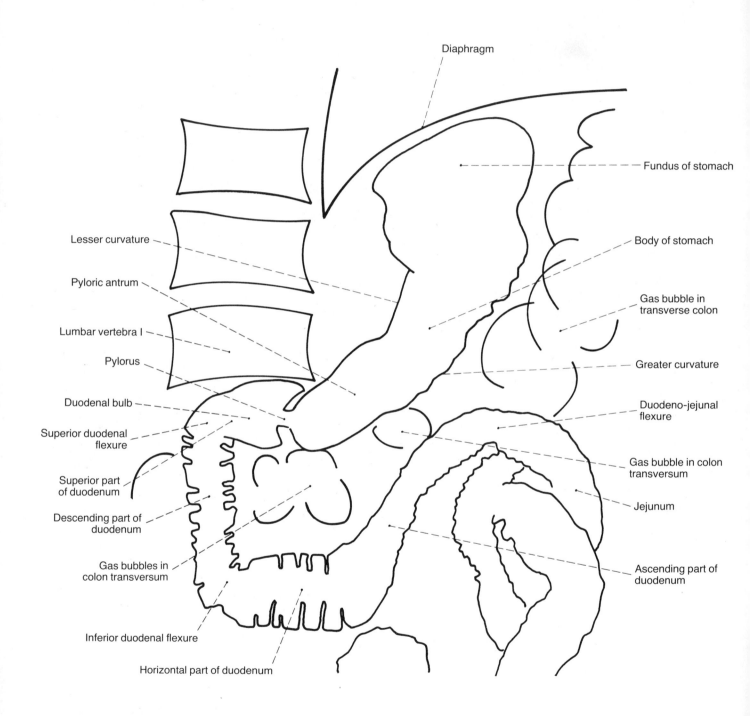

Diaphragm

Fundus of stomach

Lesser curvature

Body of stomach

Pyloric antrum

Gas bubble in
transverse colon

Lumbar vertebra I

Greater curvature

Pylorus

Duodenal bulb

Duodeno-jejunal
flexure

Superior duodenal
flexure

Gas bubble in colon
transversum

Superior part
of duodenum

Jejunum

Descending part of
duodenum

Gas bubbles in
colon transversum

Ascending part of
duodenum

Inferior duodenal flexure

Horizontal part of duodenum

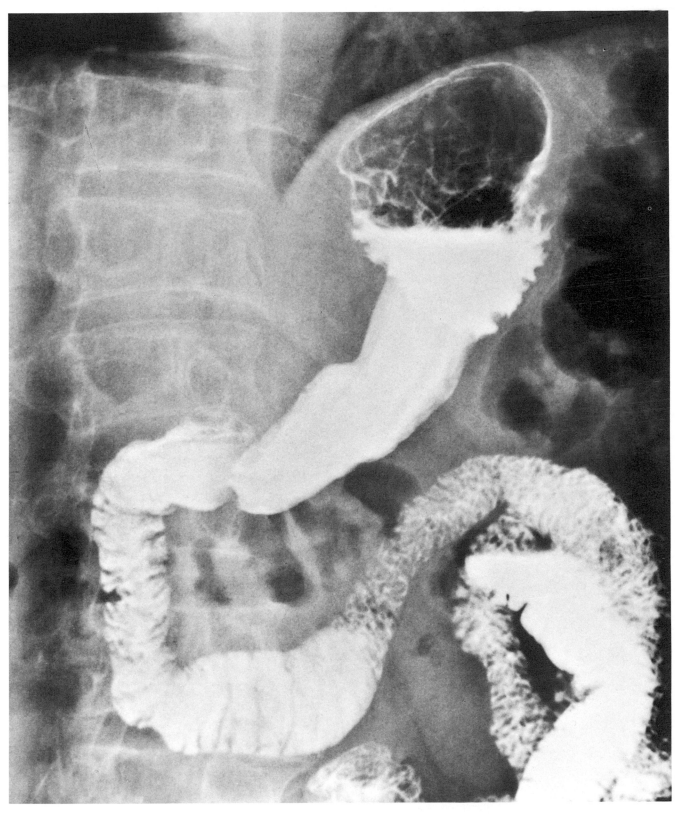

Fig. 95. Stomach (p.a. projection, patient erect)

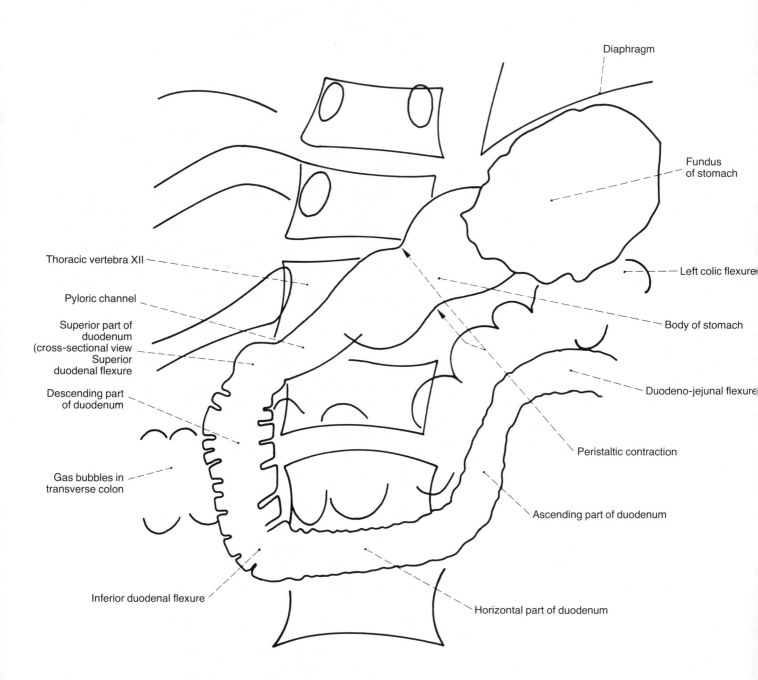

Diaphragm

Fundus
of stomach

Thoracic vertebra XII

Left colic flexure

Pyloric channel

Superior part of
duodenum
(cross-sectional view
Superior
duodenal flexure

Body of stomach

Descending part
of duodenum

Duodeno-jejunal flexure

Peristaltic contraction

Gas bubbles in
transverse colon

Ascending part of duodenum

Inferior duodenal flexure

Horizontal part of duodenum

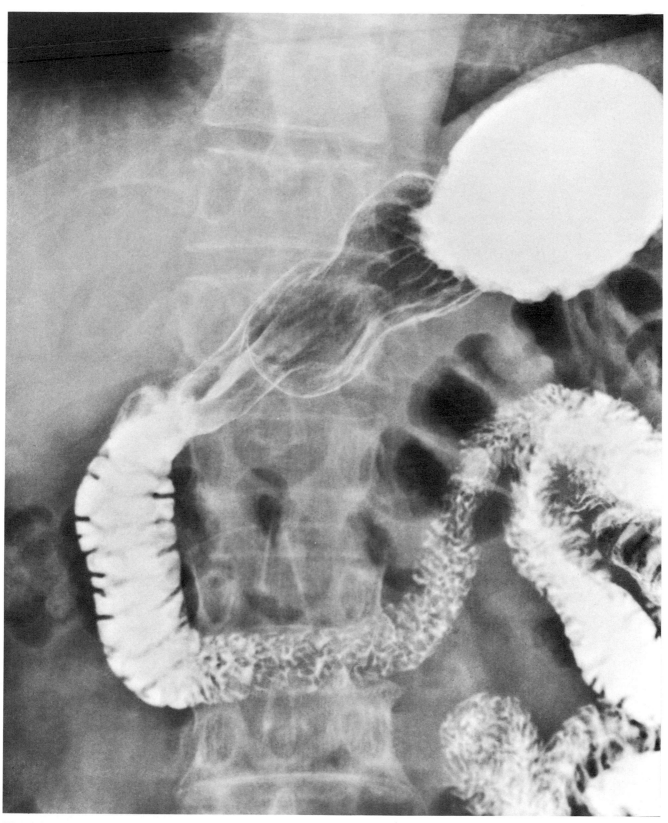

Fig. 96. Stomach, patient reclining (p.a. projection)

# Duodenum

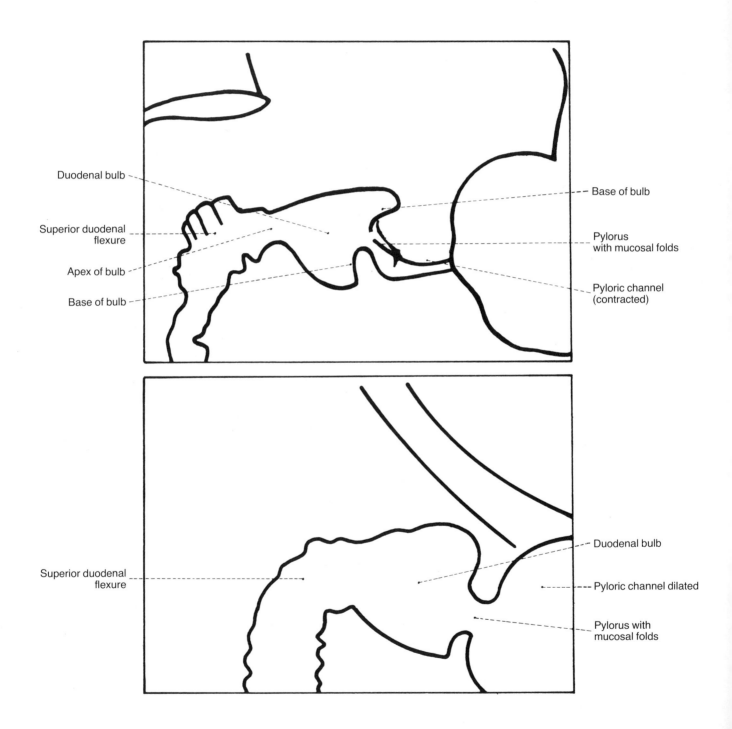

Duodenal bulb

Superior duodenal flexure

Apex of bulb

Base of bulb

Base of bulb

Pylorus with mucosal folds

Pyloric channel (contracted)

Superior duodenal flexure

Duodenal bulb

Pyloric channel dilated

Pylorus with mucosal folds

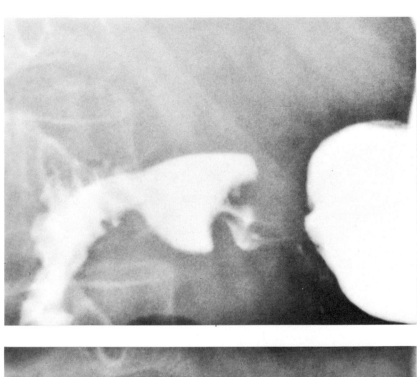

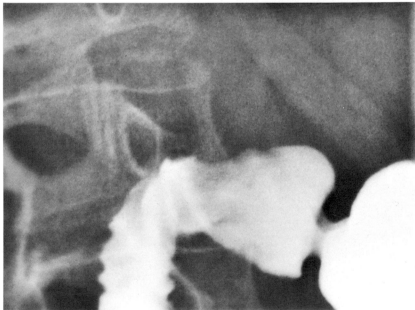

Fig. 97. Serial radiographs of bulb
(right antero-oblique projection)

# Small Intestine

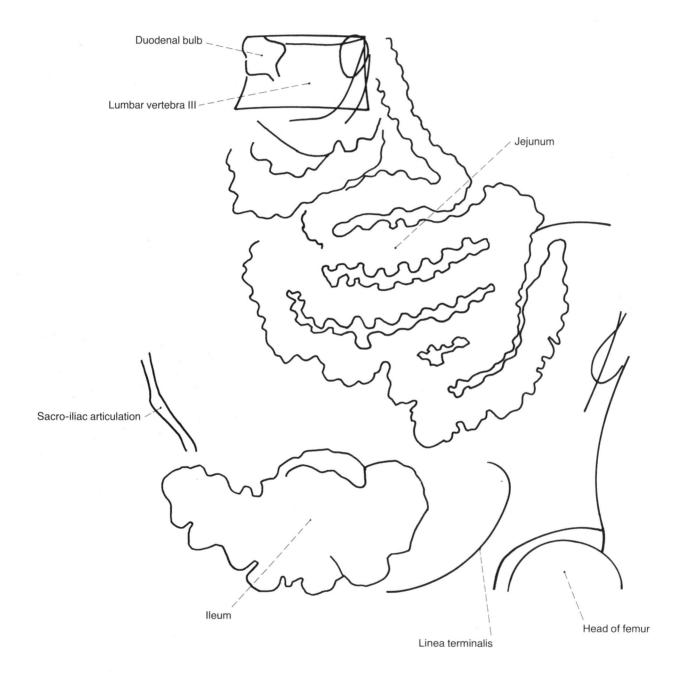

Duodenal bulb

Lumbar vertebra III

Jejunum

Sacro-iliac articulation

Ileum

Linea terminalis

Head of femur

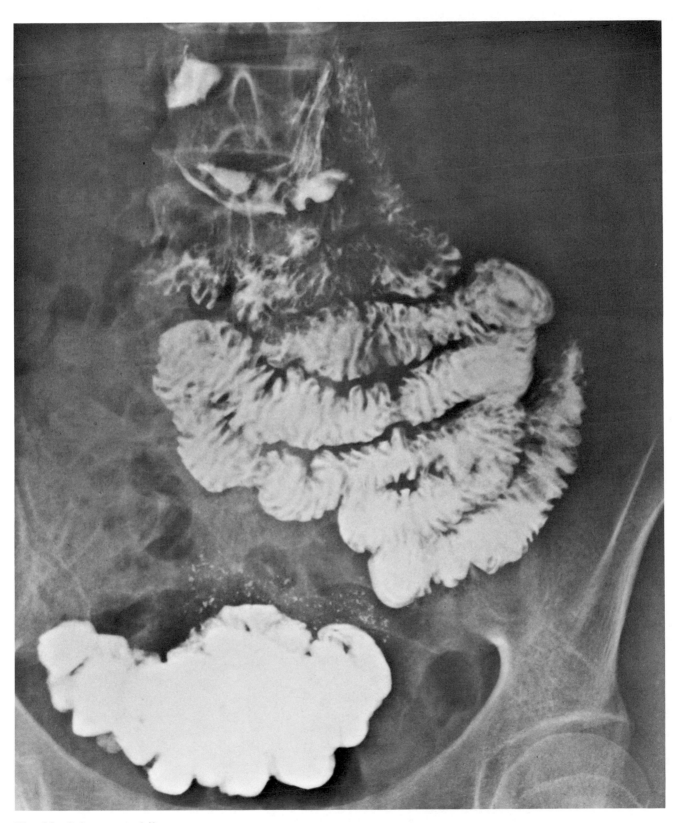

Fig. 98. Jejunum and ileum

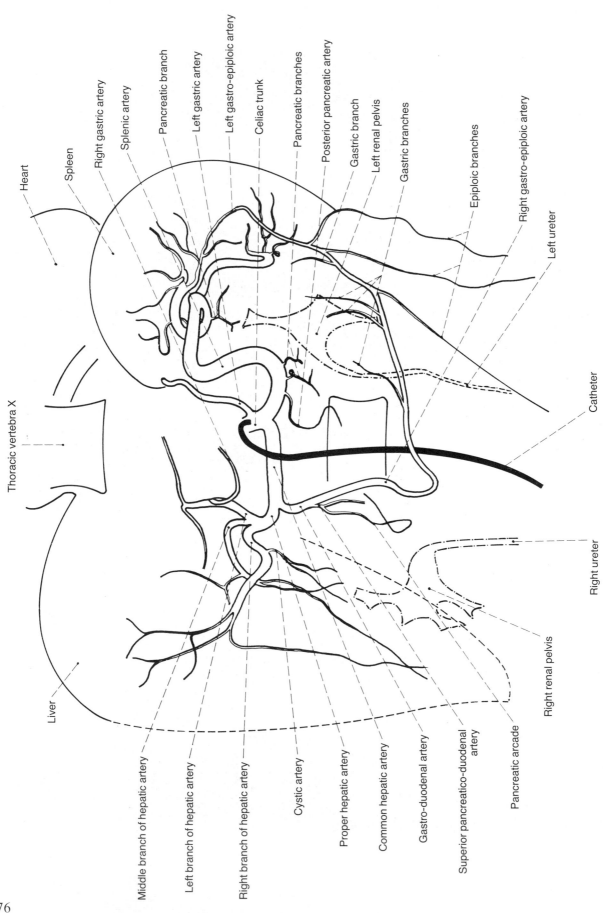

Heart

Spleen

Right gastric artery

Splenic artery

Pancreatic branch

Left gastric artery

Left gastro-epiploic artery

Celiac trunk

Pancreatic branches

Posterior pancreatic artery

Gastric branch

Left renal pelvis

Gastric branches

Epiploic branches

Right gastro-epiploic artery

Left ureter

Catheter

Thoracic vertebra X

Liver

Middle branch of hepatic artery

Left branch of hepatic artery

Right branch of hepatic artery

Cystic artery

Proper hepatic artery

Common hepatic artery

Gastro-duodenal artery

Superior pancreatico-duodenal artery

Pancreatic arcade

Right renal pelvis

Right ureter

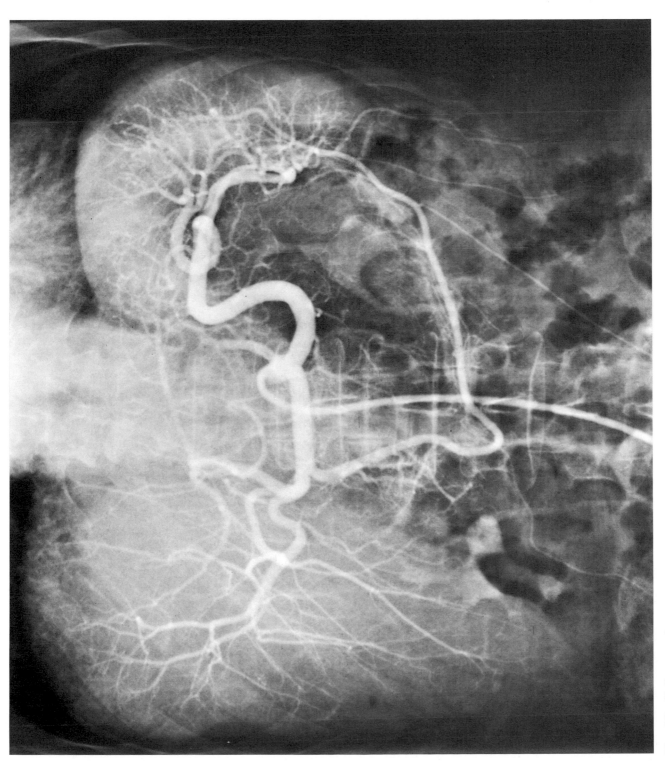

Fig. 99. Celiac arteriogram

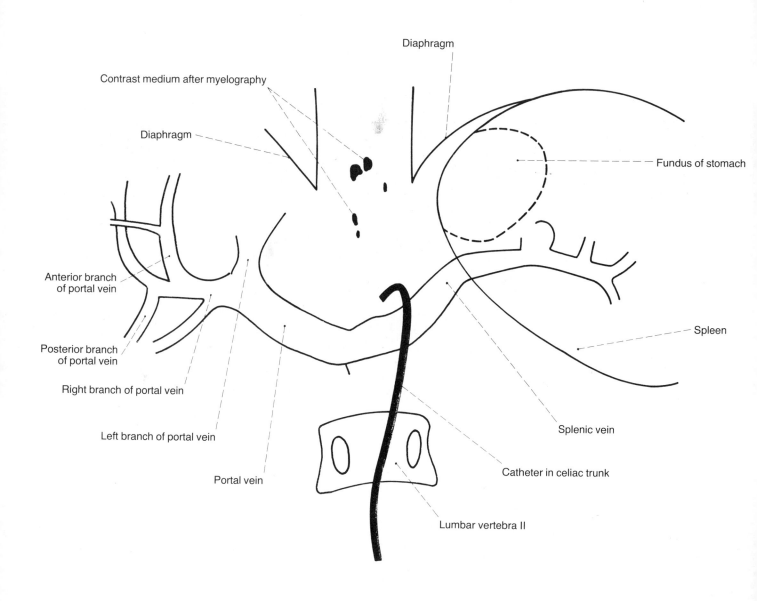

Diaphragm

Contrast medium after myelography

Diaphragm

Fundus of stomach

Anterior branch
of portal vein

Posterior branch
of portal vein

Right branch of portal vein

Left branch of portal vein

Portal vein

Spleen

Splenic vein

Catheter in celiac trunk

Lumbar vertebra II

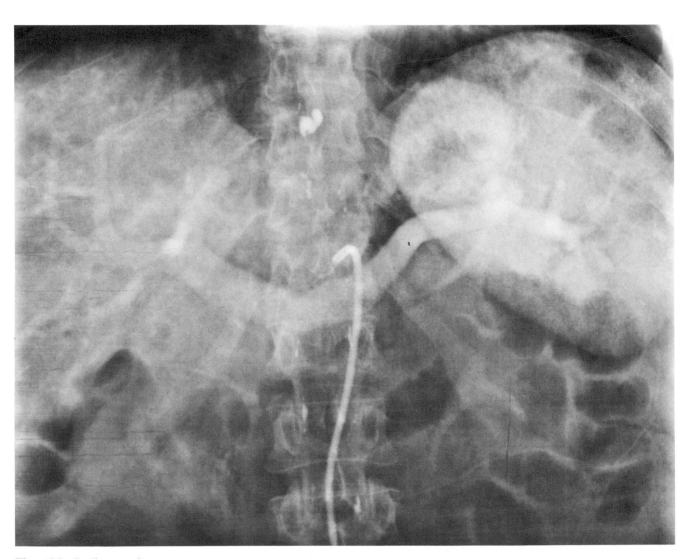

Fig. 100. Indirect splenoportogram

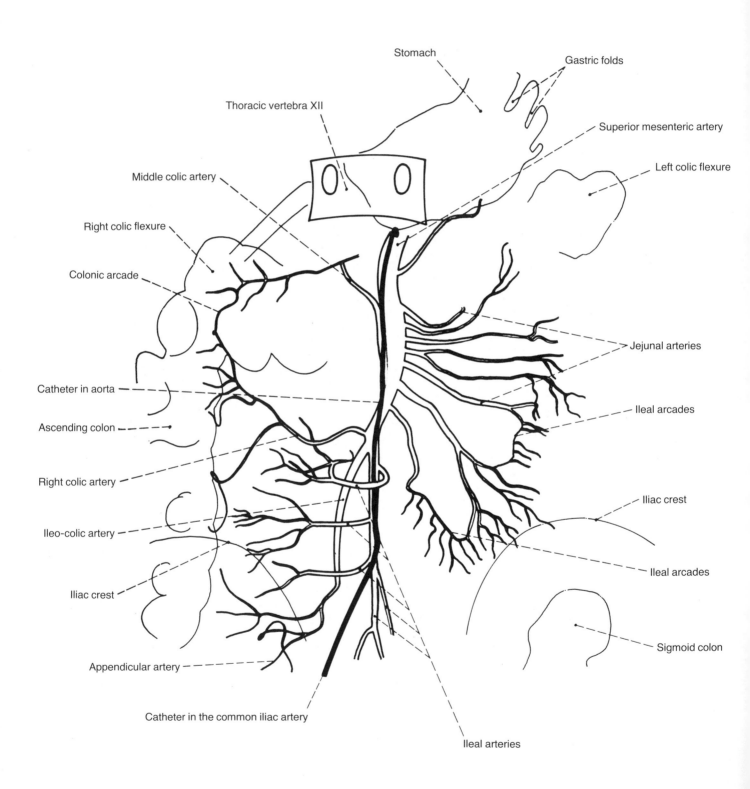

Stomach

Gastric folds

Thoracic vertebra XII

Superior mesenteric artery

Left colic flexure

Middle colic artery

Right colic flexure

Colonic arcade

Jejunal arteries

Catheter in aorta

Ileal arcades

Ascending colon

Right colic artery

Iliac crest

Ileo-colic artery

Ileal arcades

Iliac crest

Sigmoid colon

Appendicular artery

Catheter in the common iliac artery

Ileal arteries

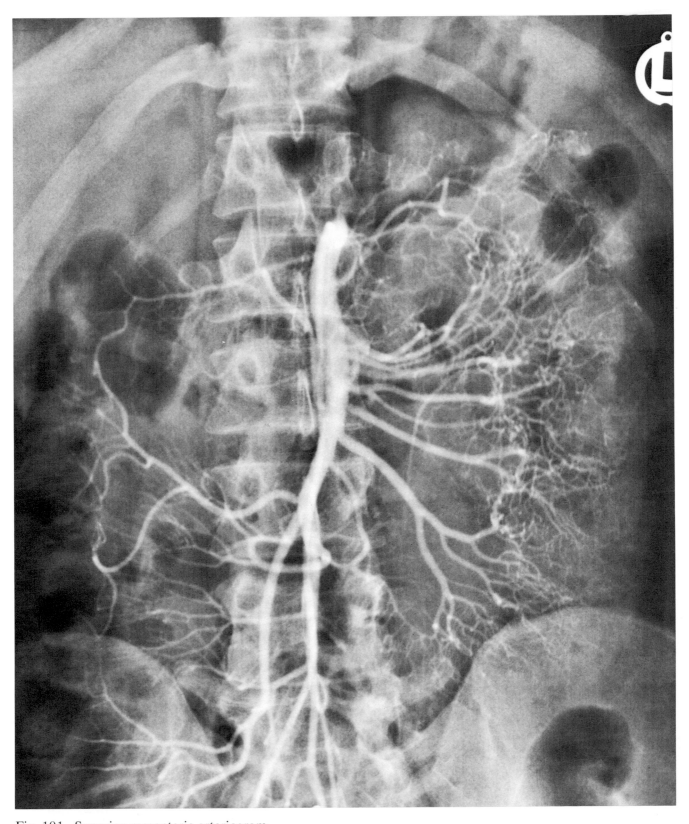

Fig. 101. Superior mesenteric arteriogram

# Inferior Mesenteric Artery

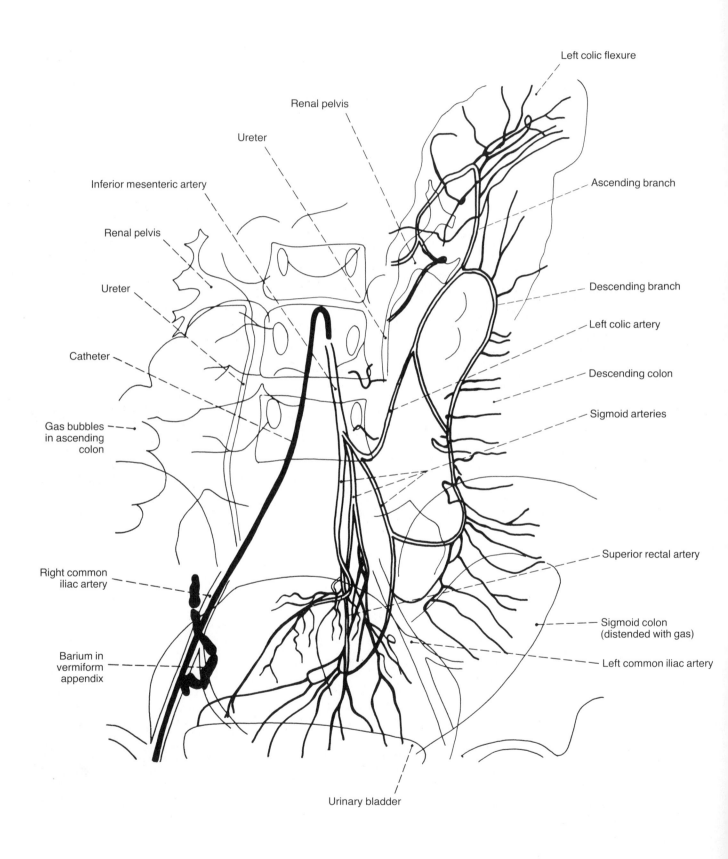

Left colic flexure

Renal pelvis

Ureter

Inferior mesenteric artery

Renal pelvis

Ureter

Catheter

Gas bubbles in ascending colon

Right common iliac artery

Barium in vermiform appendix

Ascending branch

Descending branch

Left colic artery

Descending colon

Sigmoid arteries

Superior rectal artery

Sigmoid colon (distended with gas)

Left common iliac artery

Urinary bladder

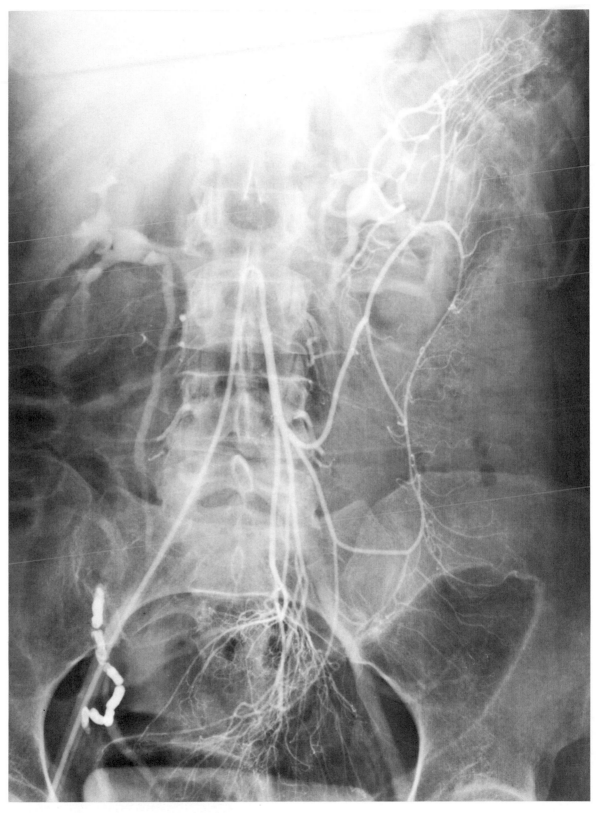

Fig. 102. Inferior mesenteric arteriogram

# Colon

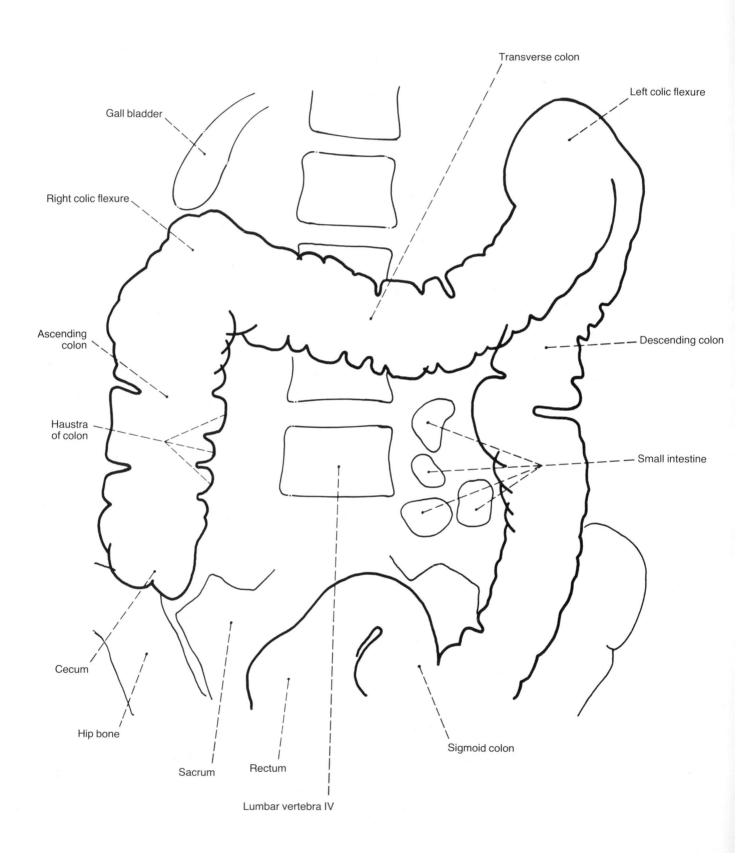

Gall bladder

Transverse colon

Left colic flexure

Right colic flexure

Ascending
colon

Descending colon

Haustra
of colon

Small intestine

Cecum

Hip bone

Sigmoid colon

Sacrum

Rectum

Lumbar vertebra IV

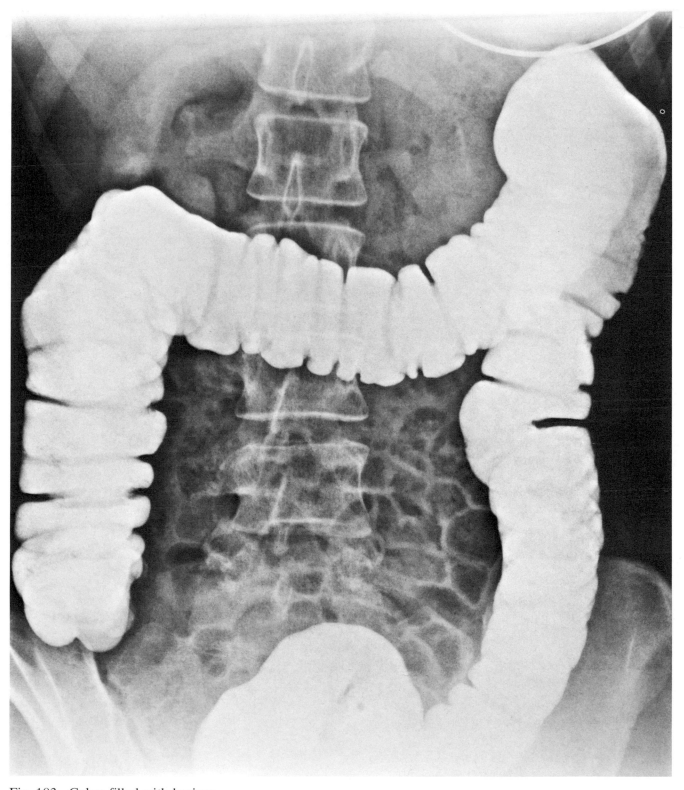

Fig. 103. Colon filled with barium

# Colon

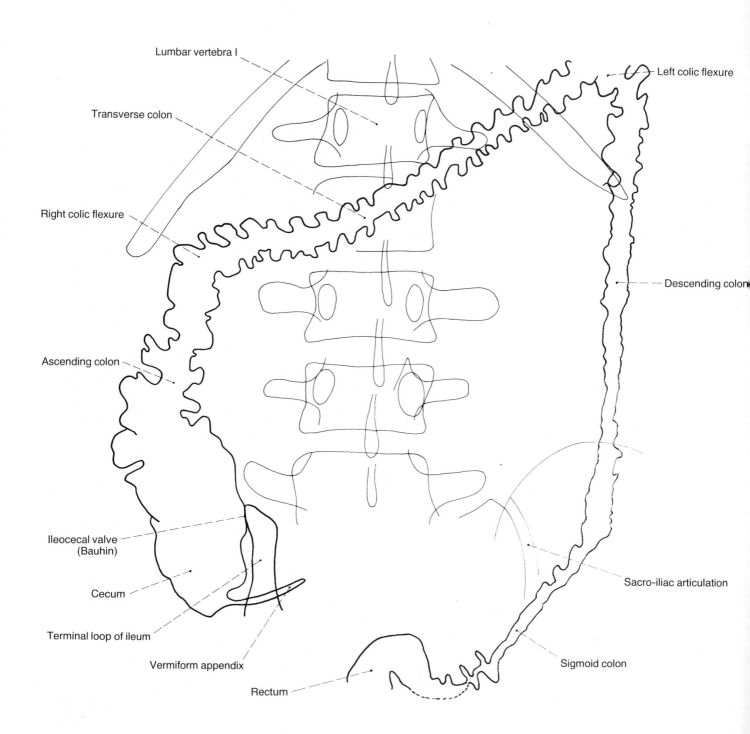

Lumbar vertebra I

Transverse colon

Right colic flexure

Ascending colon

Ileocecal valve
(Bauhin)

Cecum

Terminal loop of ileum

Vermiform appendix

Rectum

Left colic flexure

Descending colon

Sacro-iliac articulation

Sigmoid colon

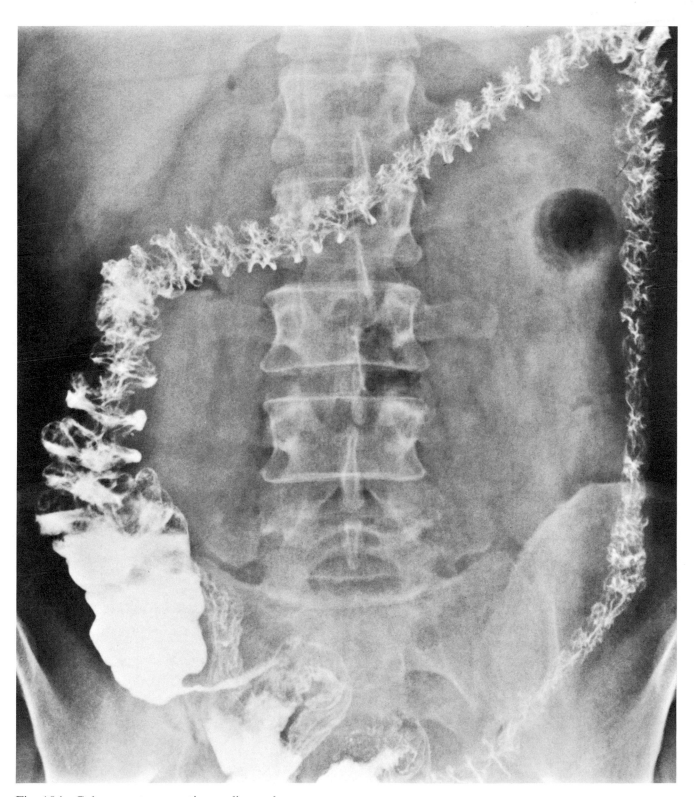

Fig. 104. Colon, post-evacuation radiograph

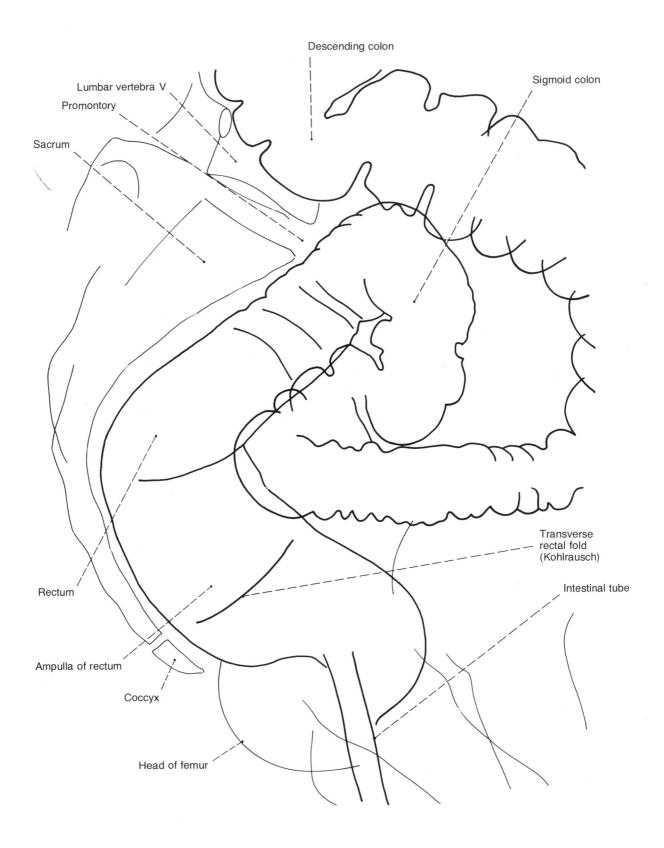

Descending colon

Sigmoid colon

Lumbar vertebra V

Promontory

Sacrum

Transverse
rectal fold
(Kohlrausch)

Rectum

Intestinal tube

Ampulla of rectum

Coccyx

Head of femur

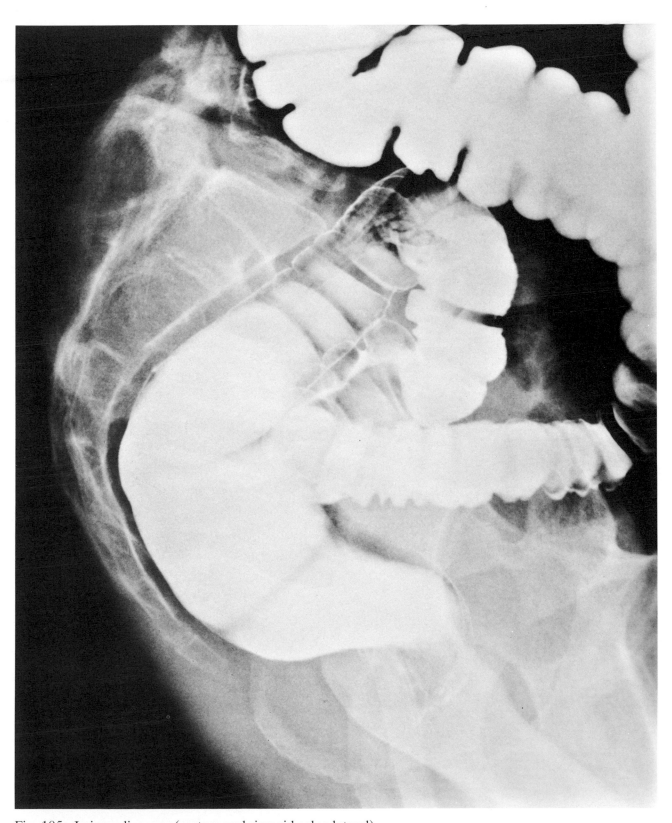

Fig. 105.  Irrigoradioscopy (rectum and sigmoid colon lateral)

# Colon

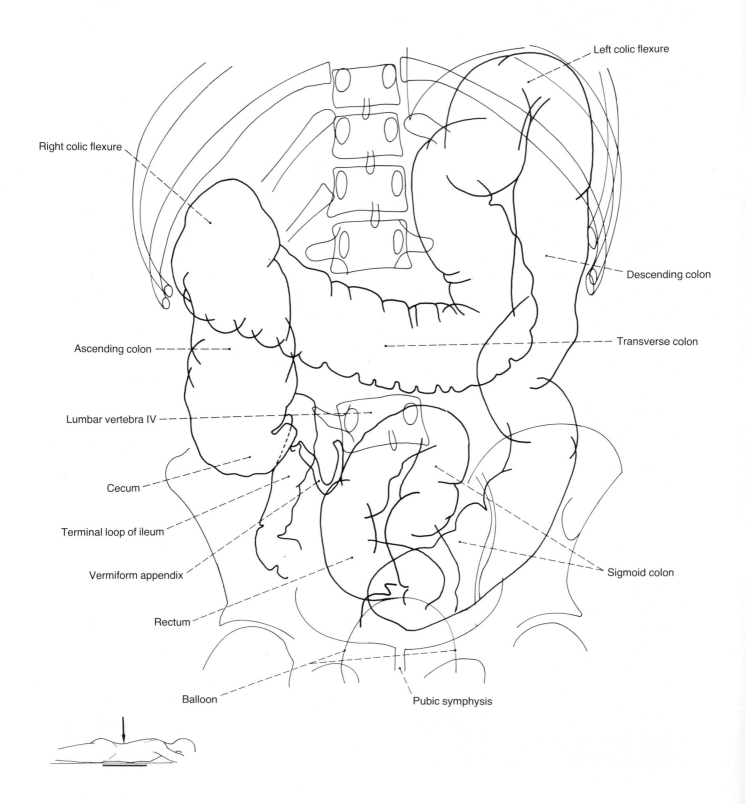

Right colic flexure

Left colic flexure

Descending colon

Ascending colon

Transverse colon

Lumbar vertebra IV

Cecum

Terminal loop of ileum

Vermiform appendix

Sigmoid colon

Rectum

Balloon

Pubic symphysis

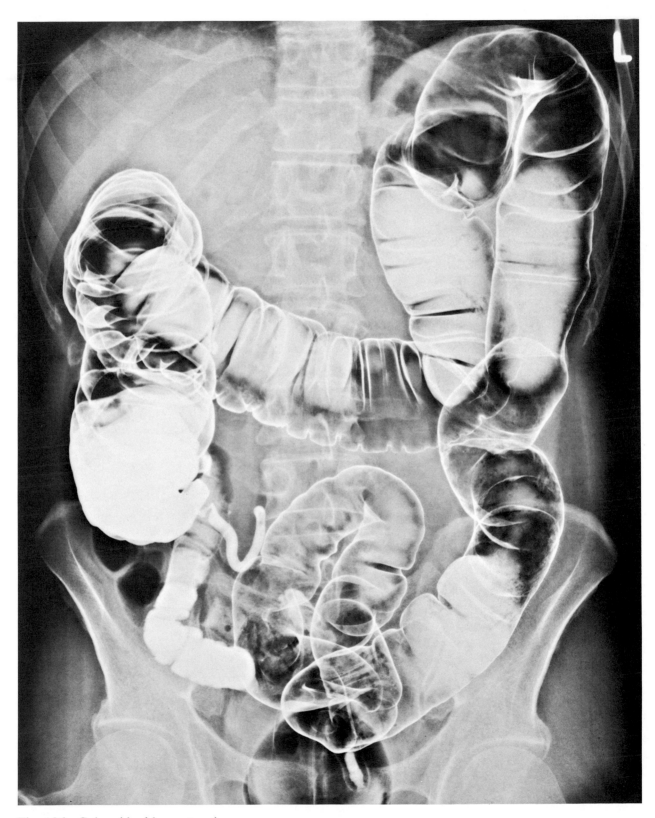

Fig. 106. Colon (double contrast)

# Biliary Tract

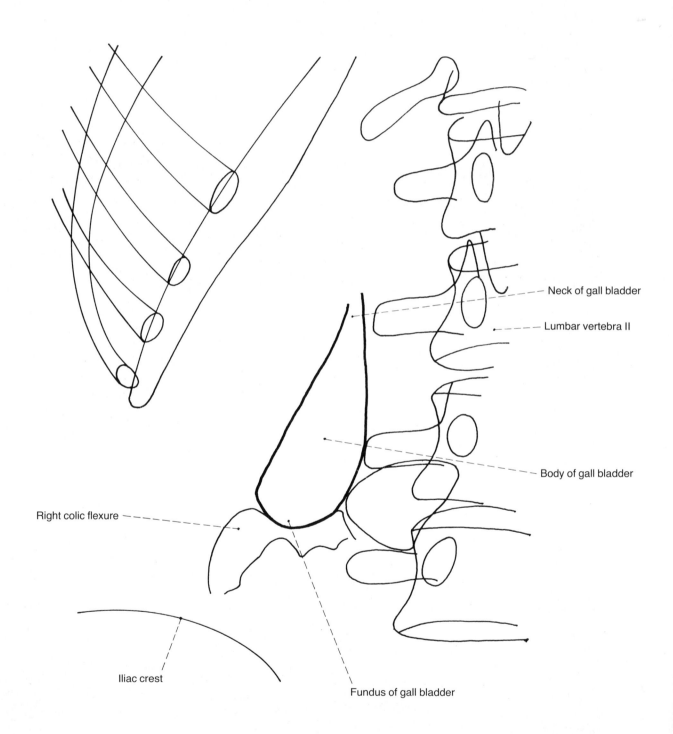

Neck of gall bladder

Lumbar vertebra II

Body of gall bladder

Right colic flexure

Fundus of gall bladder

Iliac crest

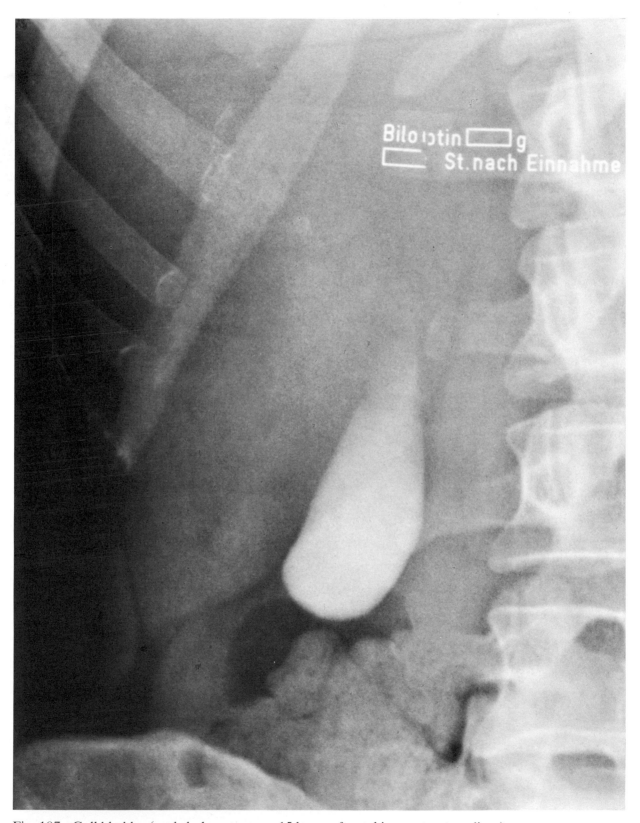

Fig. 107. Gall bladder (oral cholecystogram, 15 hours after taking contrast medium)

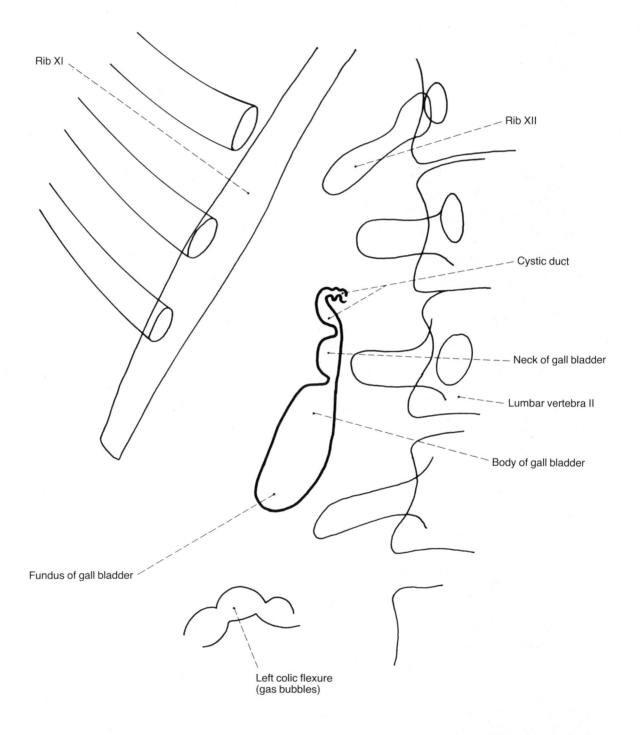

Rib XI

Rib XII

Cystic duct

Neck of gall bladder

Lumbar vertebra II

Body of gall bladder

Fundus of gall bladder

Left colic flexure
(gas bubbles)

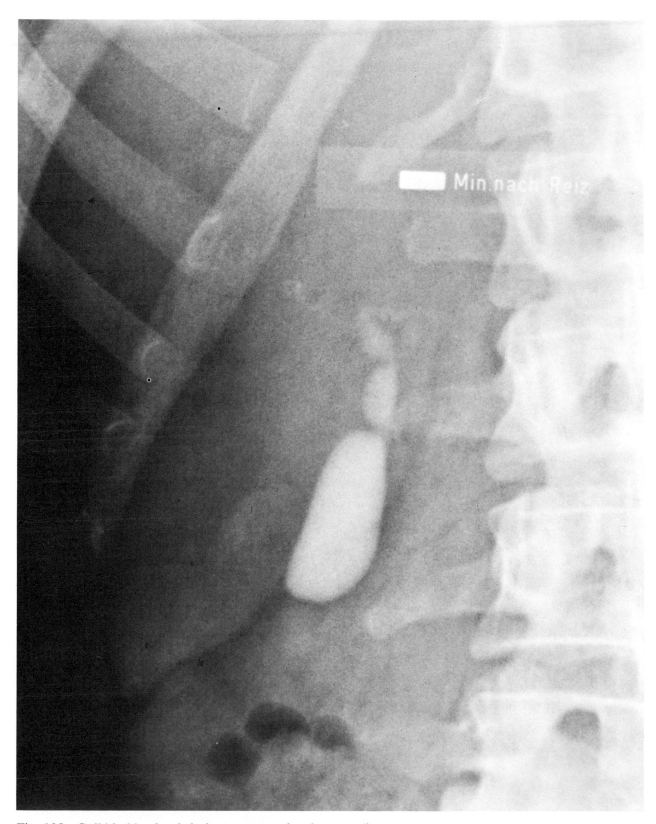

Fig. 108. Gall bladder (oral cholecystogram after fatty meal)

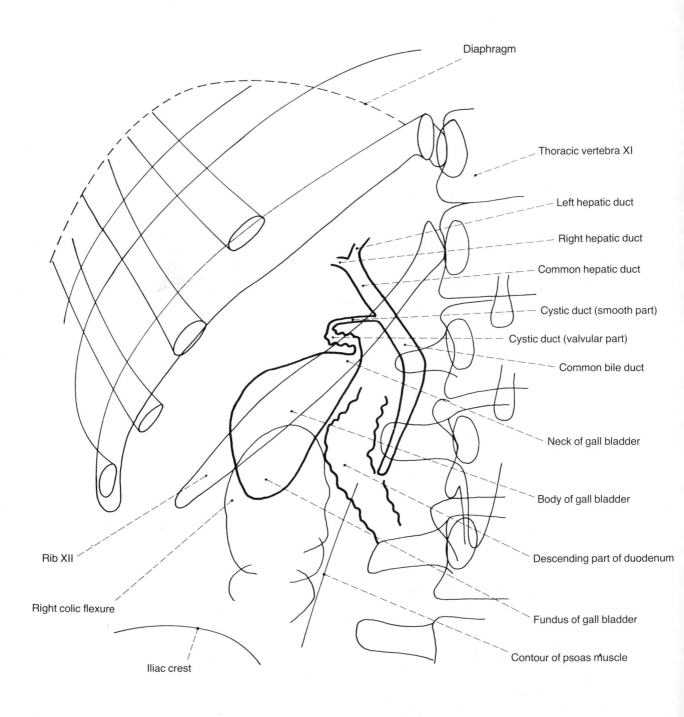

Diaphragm

Thoracic vertebra XI

Left hepatic duct

Right hepatic duct

Common hepatic duct

Cystic duct (smooth part)

Cystic duct (valvular part)

Common bile duct

Neck of gall bladder

Body of gall bladder

Descending part of duodenum

Fundus of gall bladder

Contour of psoas muscle

Rib XII

Right colic flexure

Iliac crest

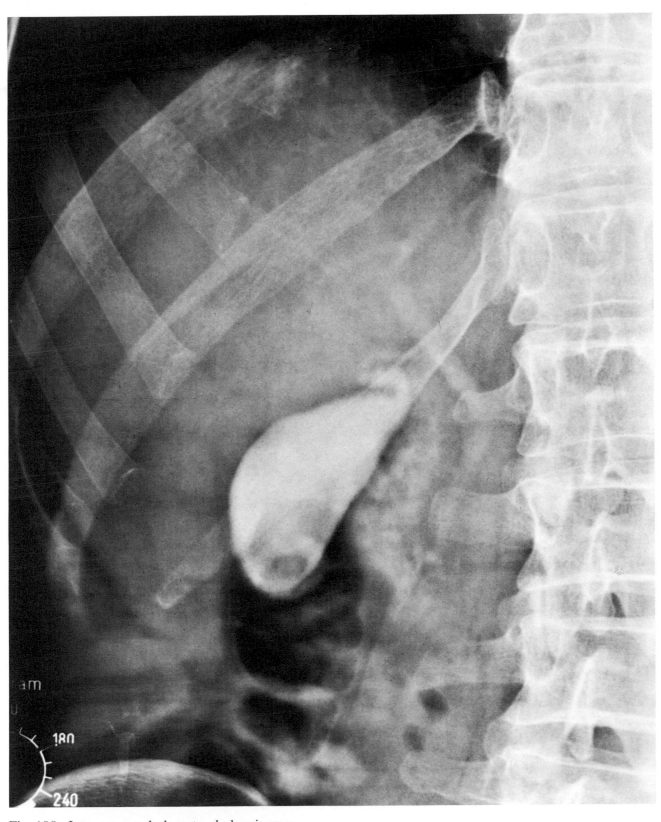

Fig. 109. Intravenous cholecysto-cholangiogram

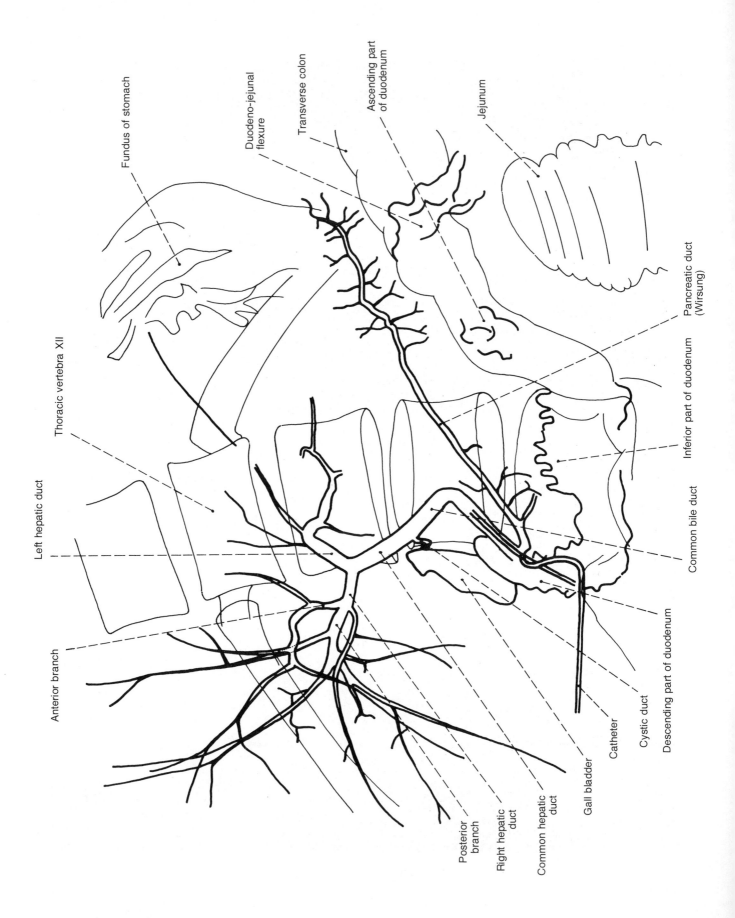

Fundus of stomach

Duodeno-jejunal flexure

Transverse colon

Ascending part of duodenum

Jejunum

Pancreatic duct (Wirsung)

Inferior part of duodenum

Common bile duct

Thoracic vertebra XII

Left hepatic duct

Anterior branch

Posterior branch

Right hepatic duct

Common hepatic duct

Gall bladder

Catheter

Cystic duct

Descending part of duodenum

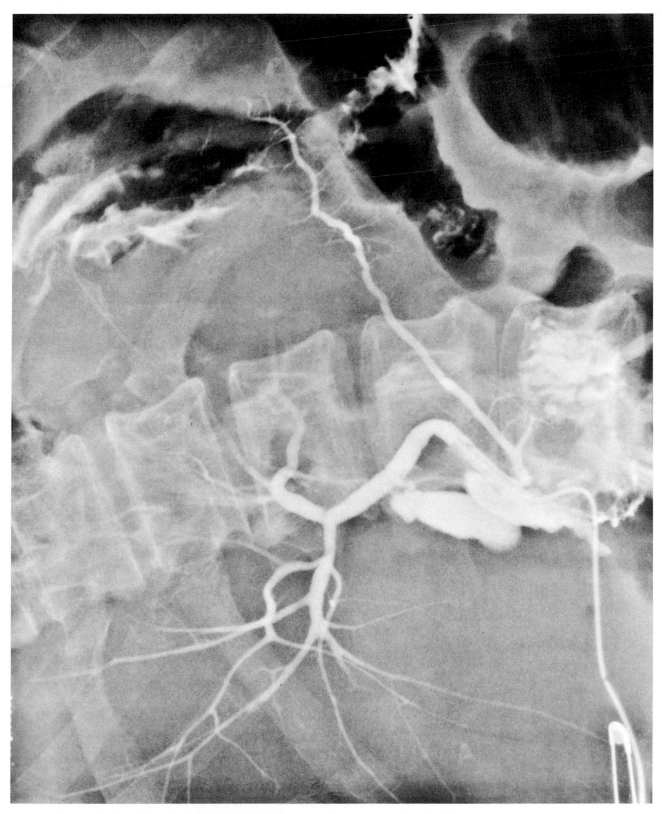

Fig. 110. Retrograde filling of the biliary tract and pancreatic duct via a T-tube and catheter

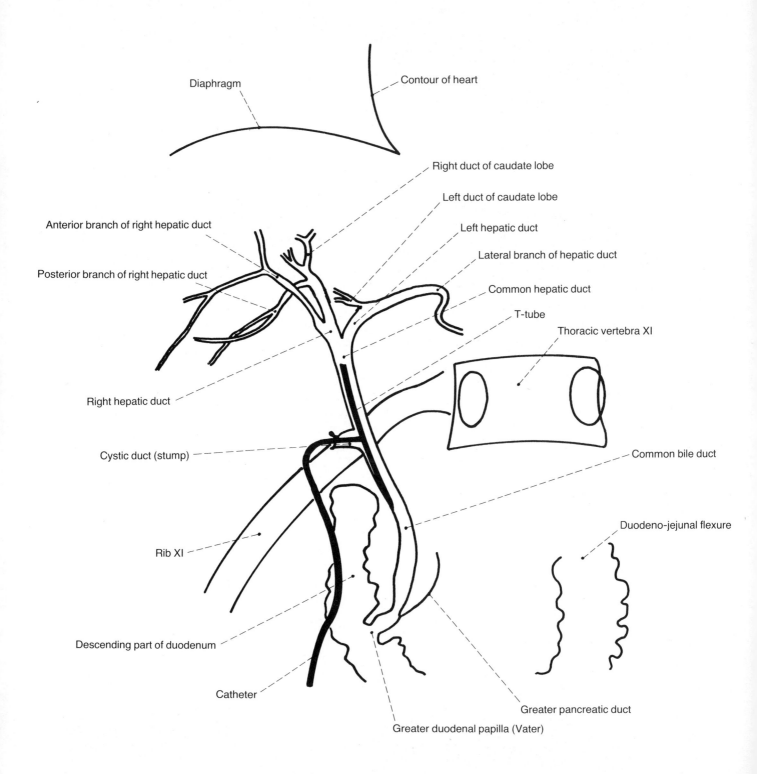

Diaphragm

Contour of heart

Right duct of caudate lobe

Left duct of caudate lobe

Anterior branch of right hepatic duct

Left hepatic duct

Lateral branch of hepatic duct

Posterior branch of right hepatic duct

Common hepatic duct

T-tube

Thoracic vertebra XI

Right hepatic duct

Cystic duct (stump)

Common bile duct

Duodeno-jejunal flexure

Rib XI

Descending part of duodenum

Catheter

Greater pancreatic duct

Greater duodenal papilla (Vater)

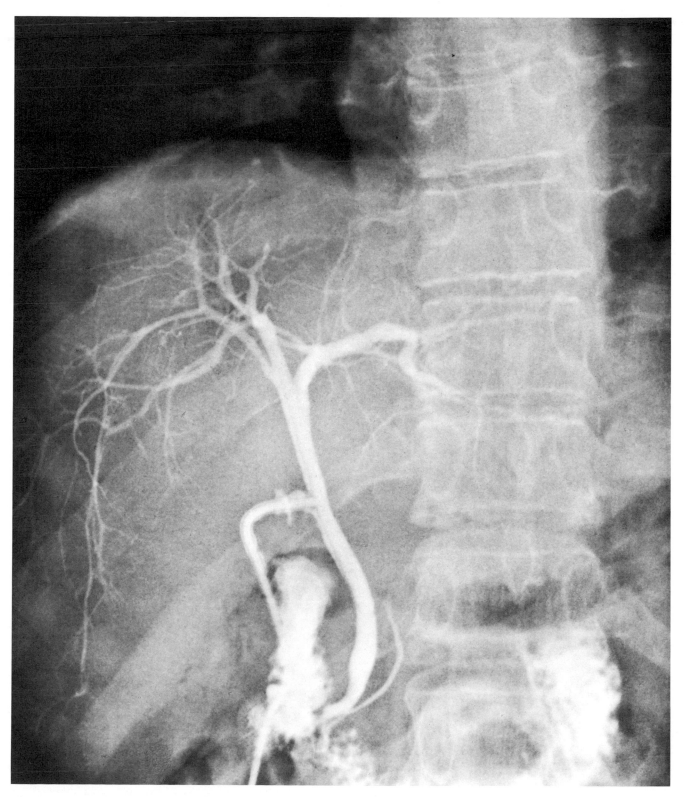

Fig. 111. Intraoperative cholangiogram (biliary tract)

# Kidneys and Urinary Tract

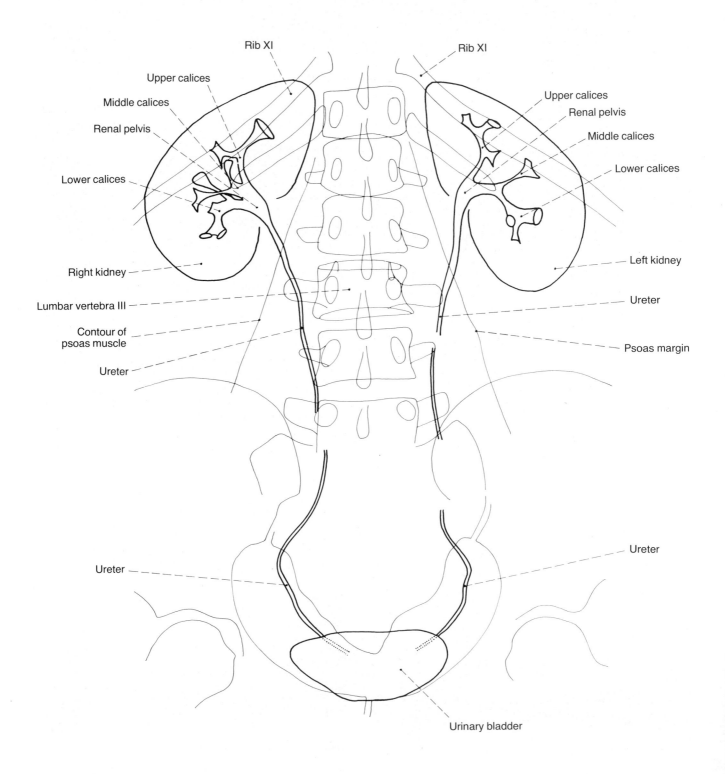

Rib XI

Rib XI

Upper calices

Middle calices

Renal pelvis

Lower calices

Right kidney

Lumbar vertebra III

Contour of
psoas muscle

Ureter

Upper calices

Renal pelvis

Middle calices

Lower calices

Left kidney

Ureter

Psoas margin

Ureter

Ureter

Urinary bladder

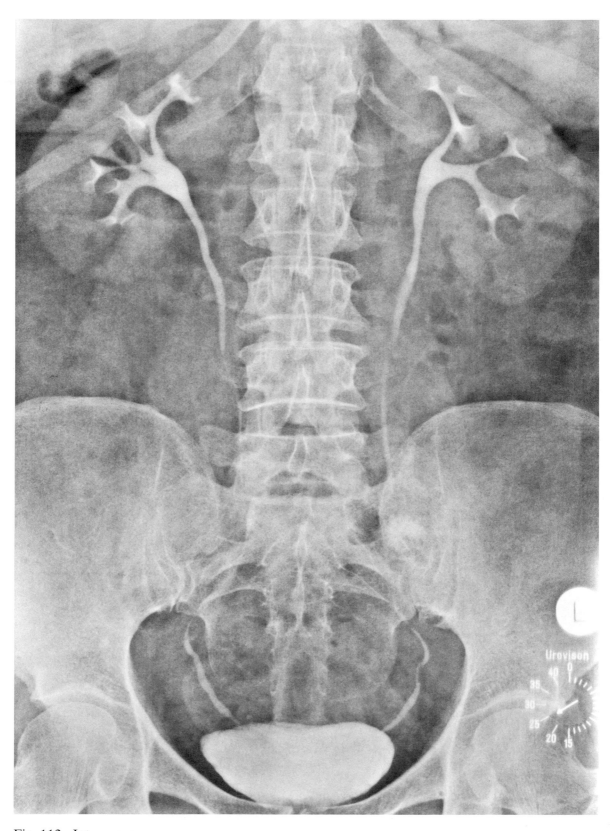

Fig. 112. Intravenous urogram

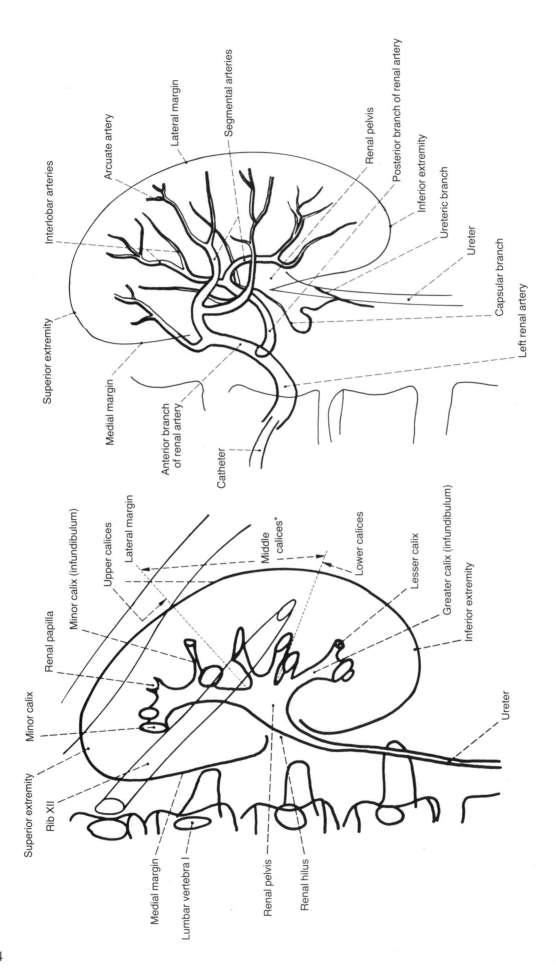

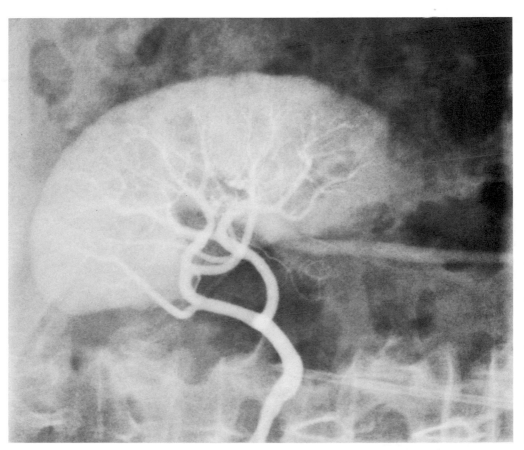

Fig. 114. Selective renal arteriogram

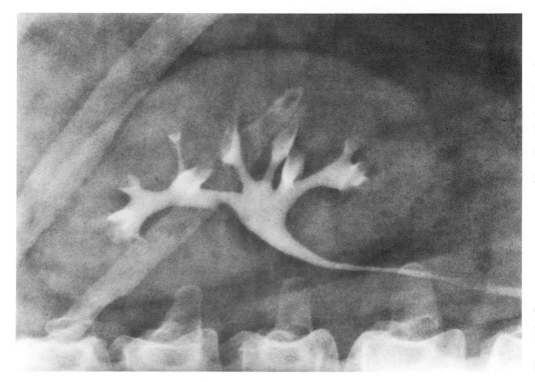

Fig. 113. Intravenous urogram (detail of left kidney)

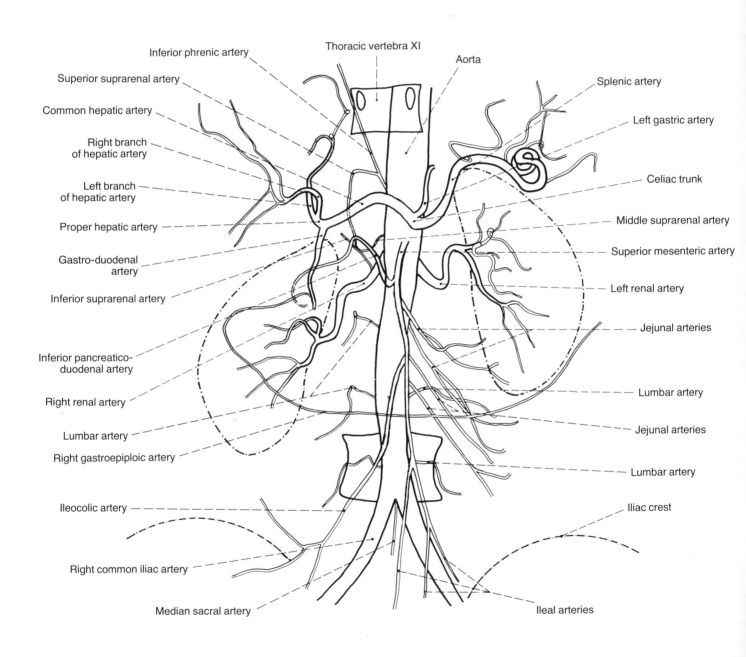

Inferior phrenic artery

Thoracic vertebra XI

Aorta

Splenic artery

Superior suprarenal artery

Left gastric artery

Common hepatic artery

Right branch
of hepatic artery

Celiac trunk

Left branch
of hepatic artery

Middle suprarenal artery

Proper hepatic artery

Superior mesenteric artery

Gastro-duodenal
artery

Left renal artery

Inferior suprarenal artery

Jejunal arteries

Inferior pancreatico-
duodenal artery

Lumbar artery

Right renal artery

Jejunal arteries

Lumbar artery

Lumbar artery

Right gastroepiploic artery

Ileocolic artery

Iliac crest

Right common iliac artery

Median sacral artery

Ileal arteries

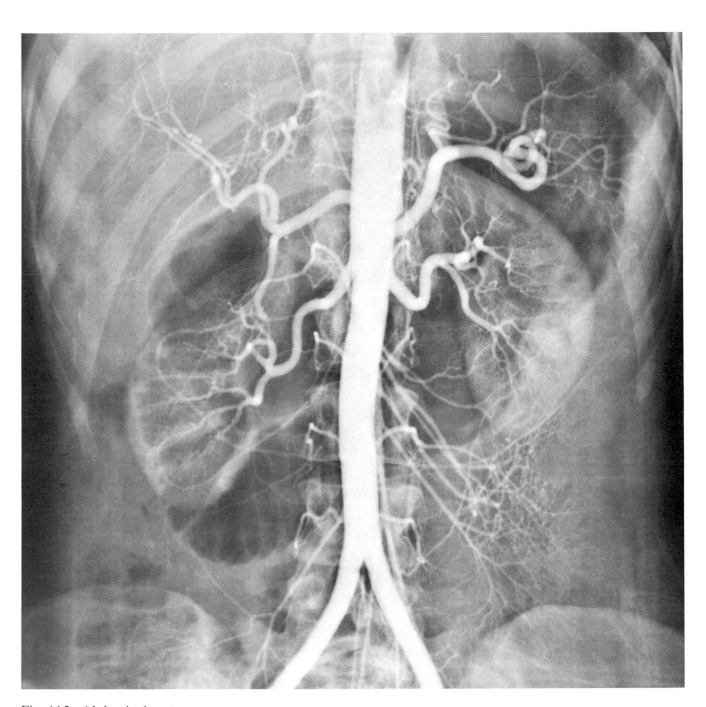

Fig. 115. Abdominal aortogram

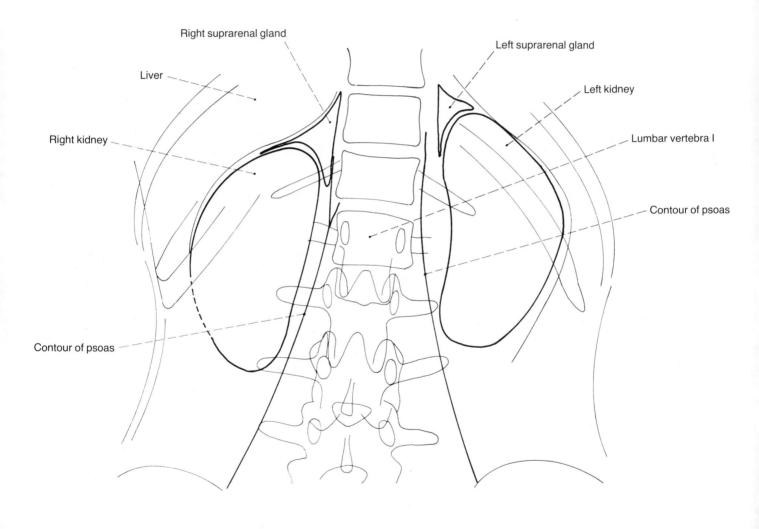

Right suprarenal gland

Left suprarenal gland

Liver

Left kidney

Right kidney

Lumbar vertebra I

Contour of psoas

Contour of psoas

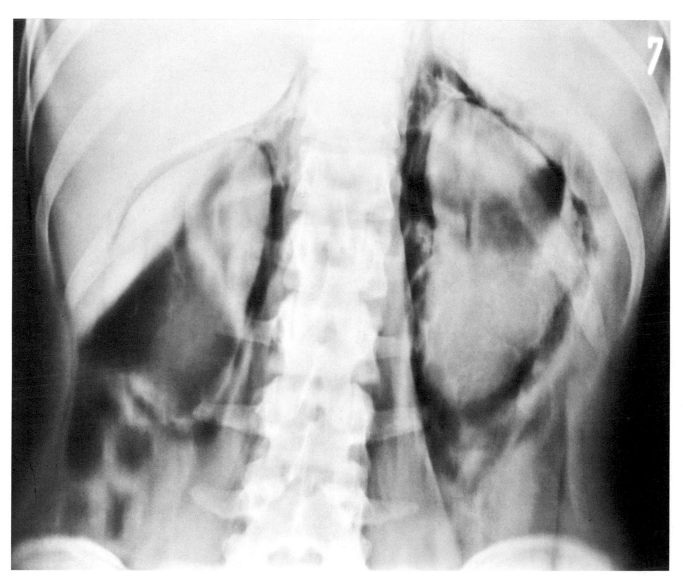

Fig. 116. Retroperitoneal air study (tomogram)

# Veins

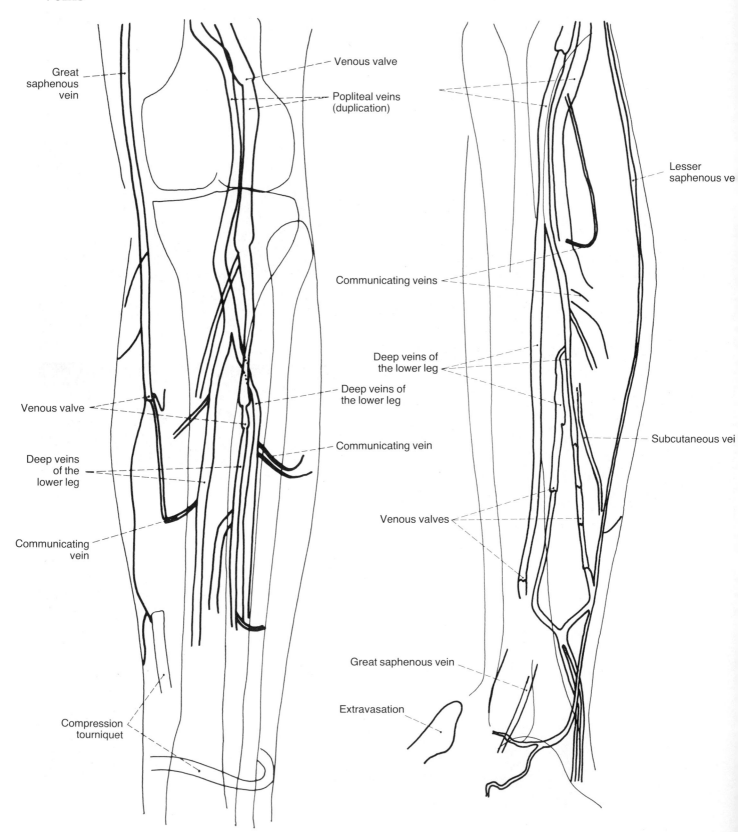

Great saphenous vein

Venous valve

Popliteal veins (duplication)

Lesser saphenous vein

Communicating veins

Deep veins of the lower leg

Venous valve

Deep veins of the lower leg

Communicating vein

Deep veins of the lower leg

Subcutaneous vein

Communicating vein

Venous valves

Compression tourniquet

Great saphenous vein

Extravasation

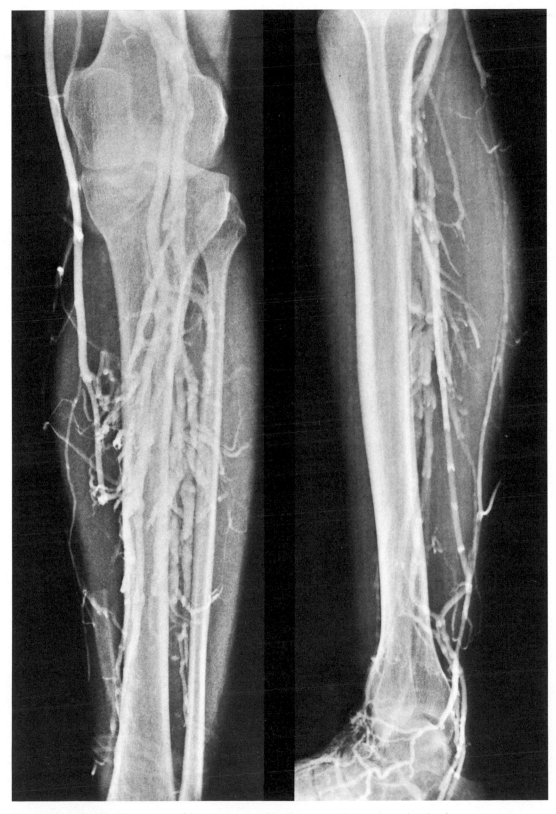

Fig. 117/118. Phlebogram of lower extremity (p.a. and lateral projection)

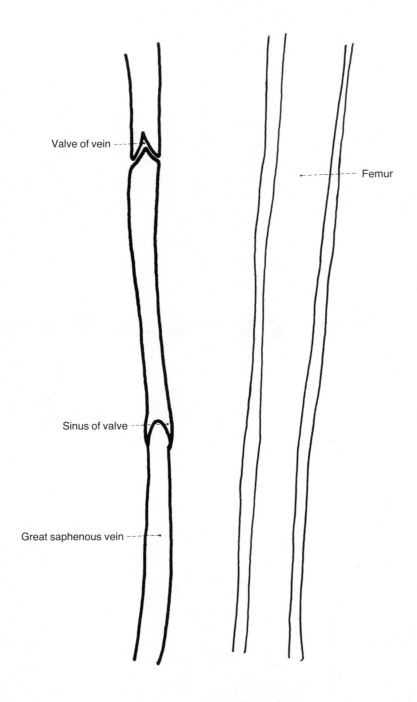

Valve of vein

Femur

Sinus of valve

Great saphenous vein

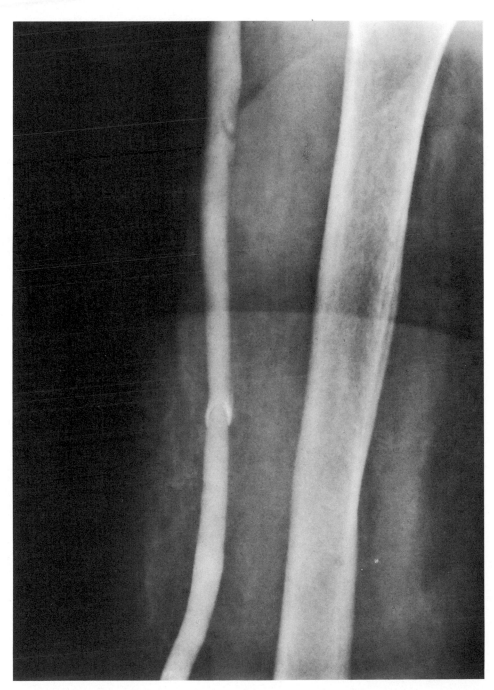

Fig. 119. Venous valve

# Lymphography

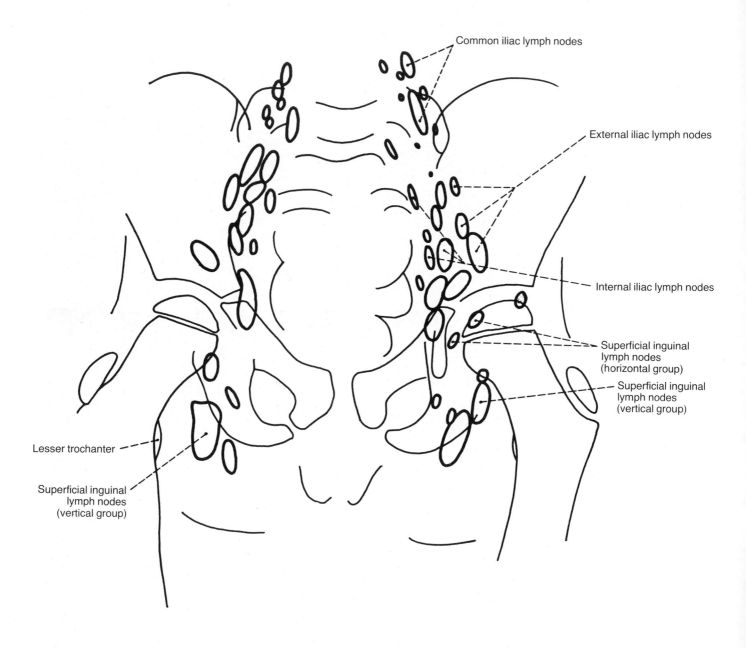

Common iliac lymph nodes

External iliac lymph nodes

Internal iliac lymph nodes

Superficial inguinal
lymph nodes
(horizontal group)

Superficial inguinal
lymph nodes
(vertical group)

Lesser trochanter

Superficial inguinal
lymph nodes
(vertical group)

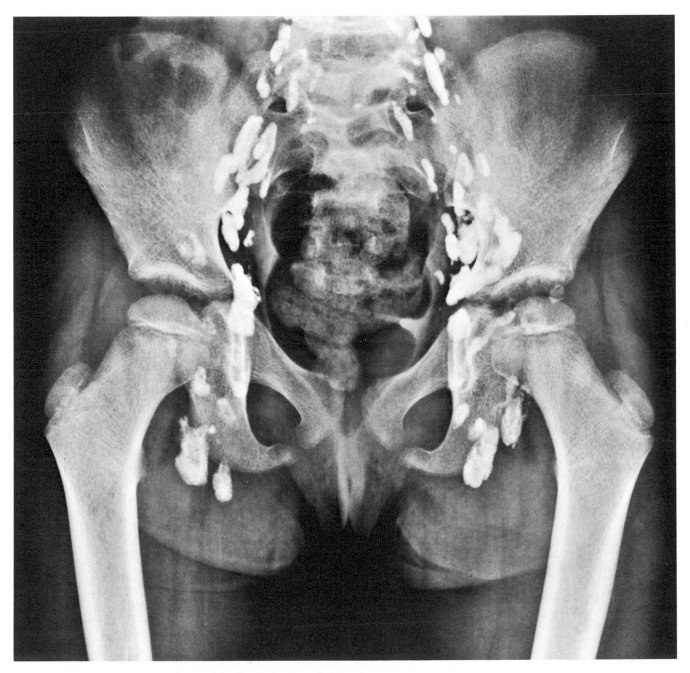

Fig. 120. Pelvic lymphogram, nodal phase (a.p. projection)

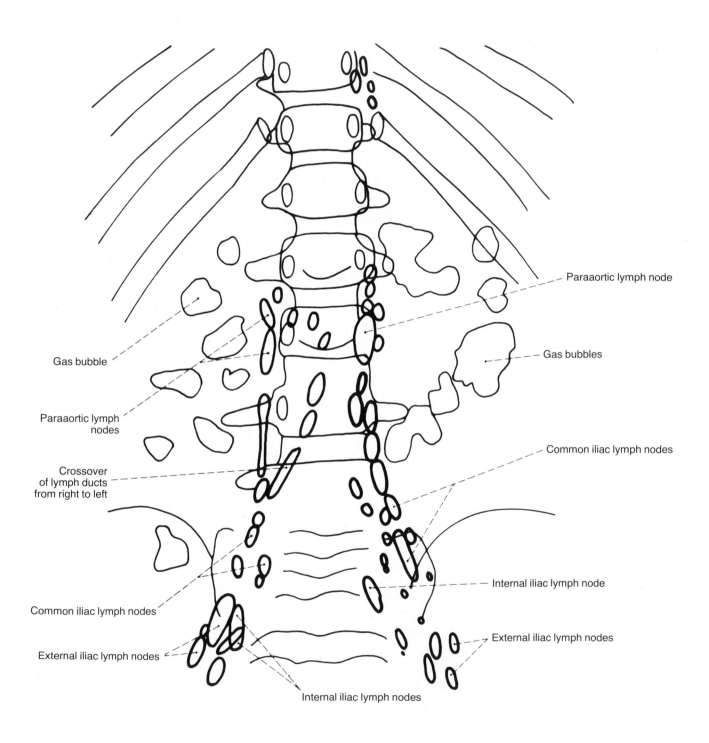

Paraaortic lymph node

Gas bubble

Gas bubbles

Paraaortic lymph
nodes

Common iliac lymph nodes

Crossover
of lymph ducts
from right to left

Internal iliac lymph node

Common iliac lymph nodes

External iliac lymph nodes

External iliac lymph nodes

Internal iliac lymph nodes

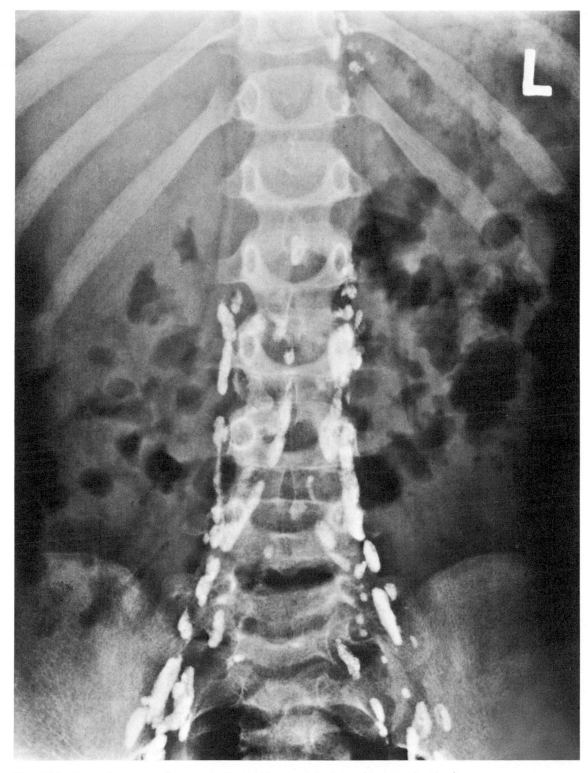

Fig. 121. Lymphogram of para-aortic region, nodal phase (a.p. projection)

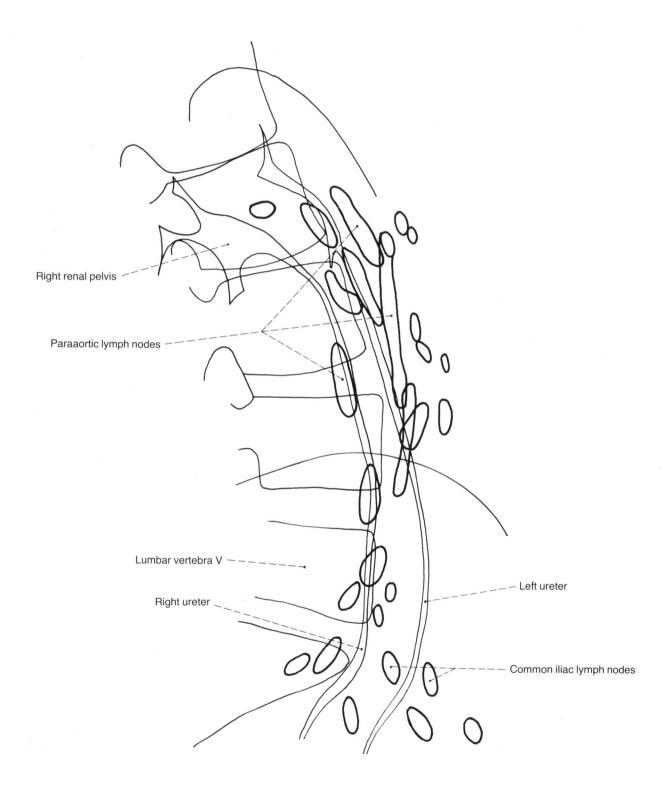

Right renal pelvis

Paraaortic lymph nodes

Lumbar vertebra V

Right ureter

Left ureter

Common iliac lymph nodes

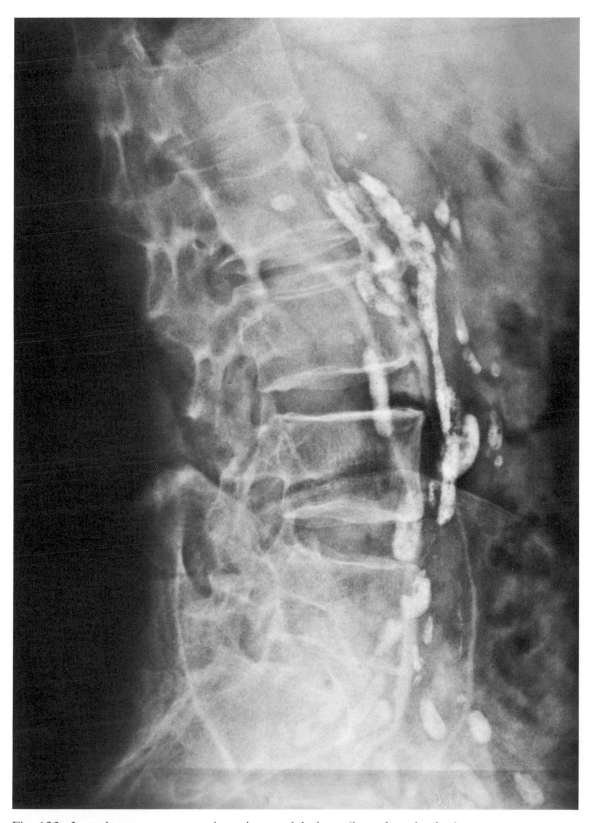

Fig. 122. Lymphogram, para-aortic region, nodal phase (lateral projection)

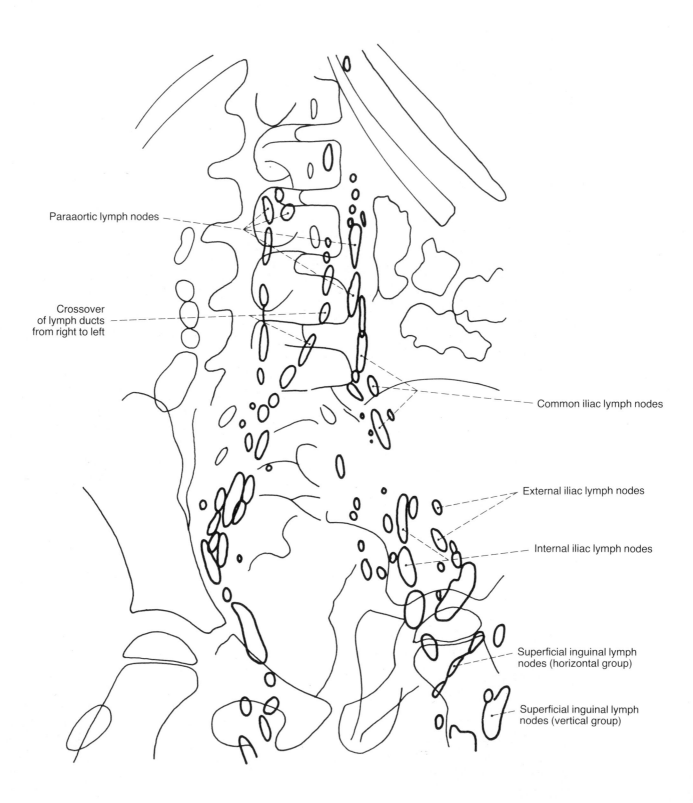

Paraaortic lymph nodes

Crossover
of lymph ducts
from right to left

Common iliac lymph nodes

External iliac lymph nodes

Internal iliac lymph nodes

Superficial inguinal lymph
nodes (horizontal group)

Superficial inguinal lymph
nodes (vertical group)

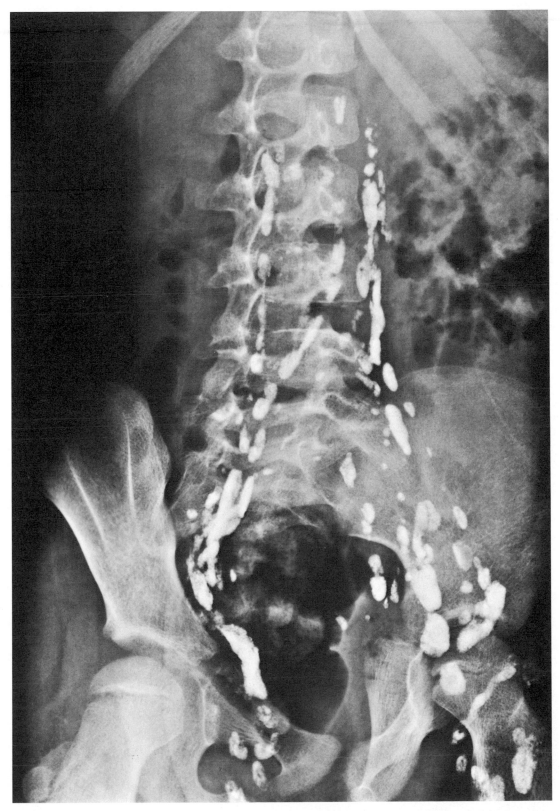

Fig. 123. Lymphogram, pelvic and para-aortic regions (oblique projection, nodal phase)

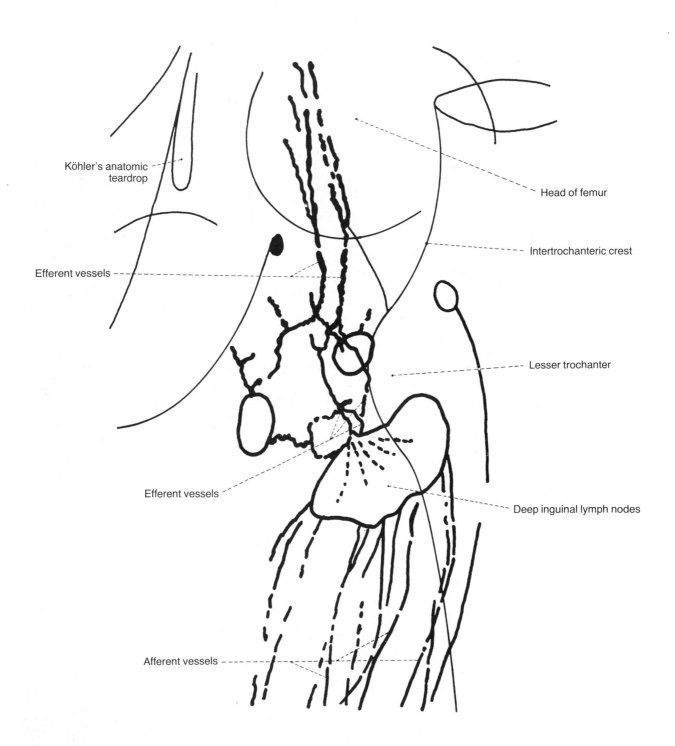

Köhler's anatomic
teardrop

Head of femur

Intertrochanteric crest

Efferent vessels

Lesser trochanter

Efferent vessels

Deep inguinal lymph nodes

Afferent vessels

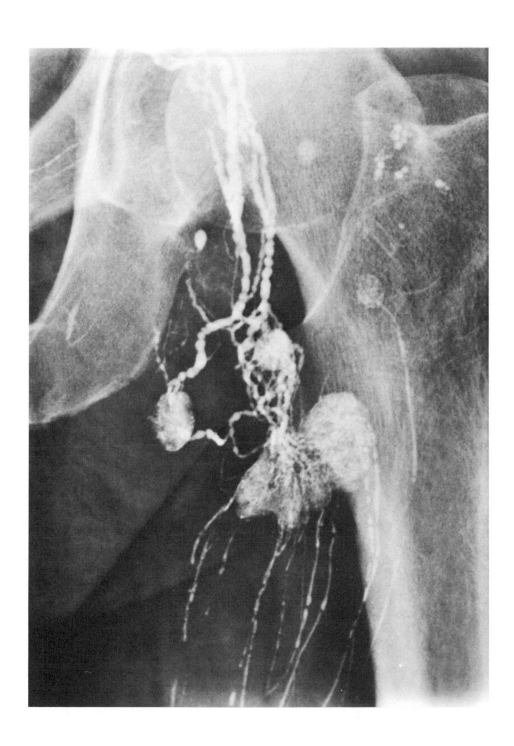

Fig. 124. Lymphogram
of inguinal lymph nodes
(vascular phase)

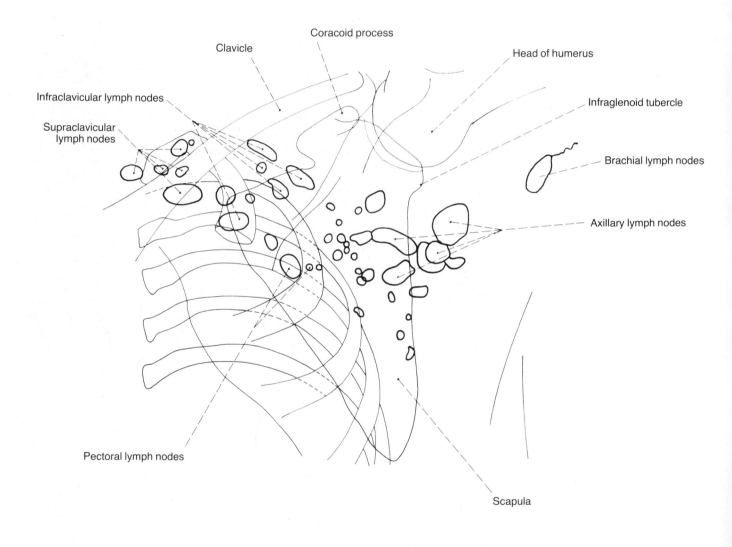

Coracoid process

Clavicle

Head of humerus

Infraclavicular lymph nodes

Infraglenoid tubercle

Supraclavicular
lymph nodes

Brachial lymph nodes

Axillary lymph nodes

Pectoral lymph nodes

Scapula

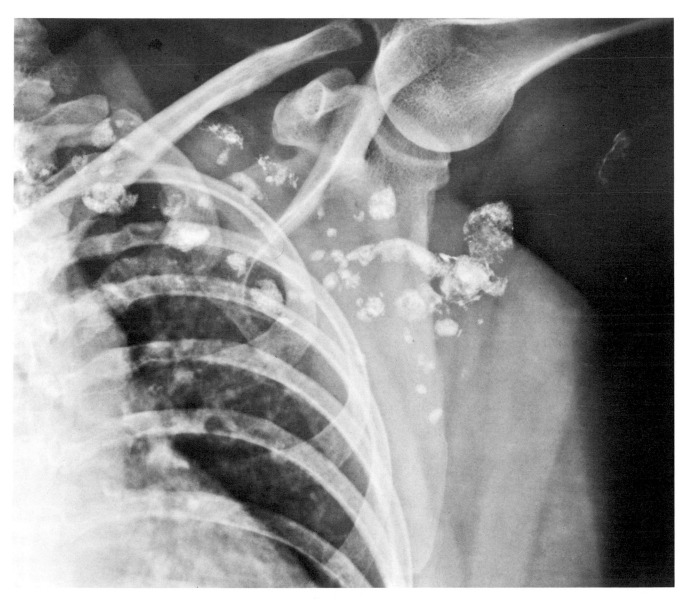

Fig. 125. Lymphogram, axillary lymph nodes (nodal phase)

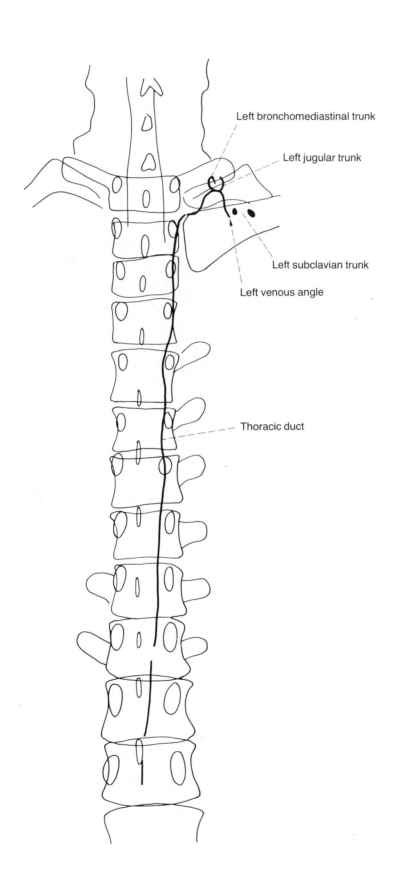

Left bronchomediastinal trunk

Left jugular trunk

Left subclavian trunk

Left venous angle

Thoracic duct

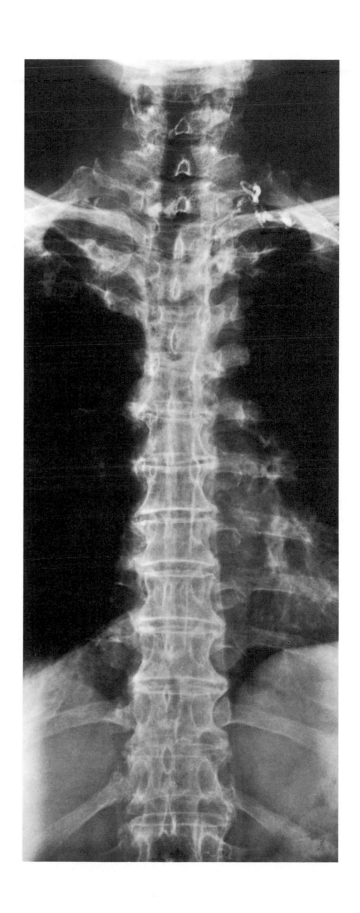

Fig. 126. Lymphogram of thoracic duct

# Gynecologic Radiography

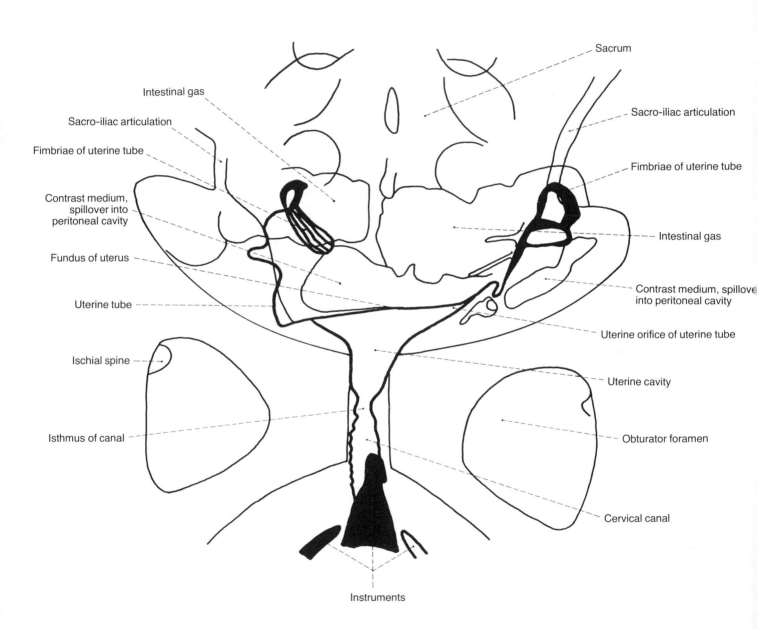

Sacrum

Intestinal gas

Sacro-iliac articulation

Sacro-iliac articulation

Fimbriae of uterine tube

Fimbriae of uterine tube

Contrast medium, spillover into peritoneal cavity

Intestinal gas

Fundus of uterus

Contrast medium, spillover into peritoneal cavity

Uterine tube

Uterine orifice of uterine tube

Ischial spine

Uterine cavity

Isthmus of canal

Obturator foramen

Cervical canal

Instruments

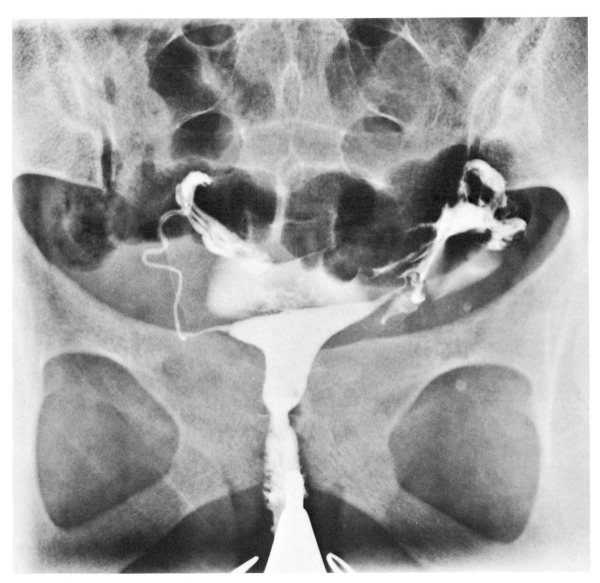

Fig. 127. Hysterosalpingogram

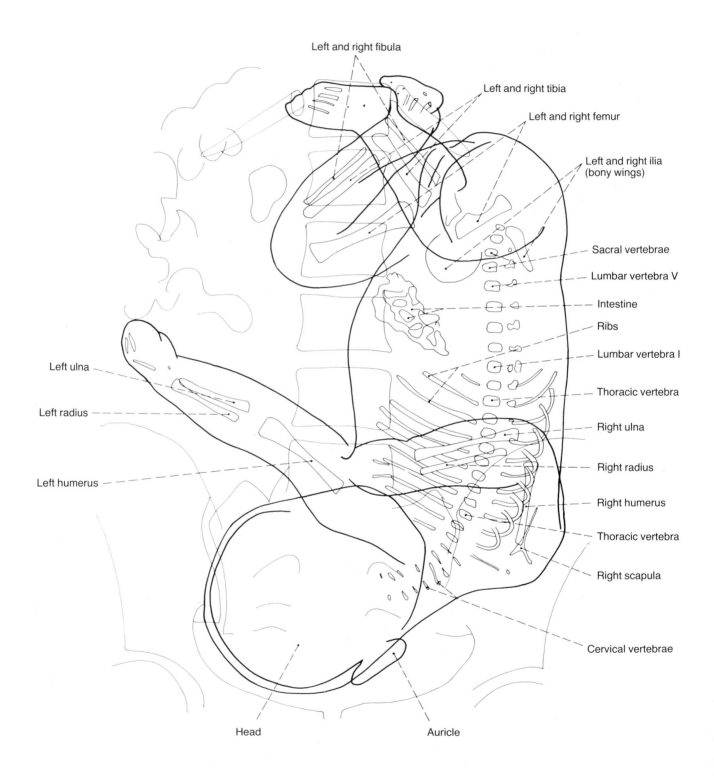

Left and right fibula

Left and right tibia

Left and right femur

Left and right ilia
(bony wings)

Sacral vertebrae

Lumbar vertebra V

Intestine

Ribs

Lumbar vertebra I

Thoracic vertebra

Left ulna

Right ulna

Left radius

Right radius

Left humerus

Right humerus

Thoracic vertebra

Right scapula

Cervical vertebrae

Head

Auricle

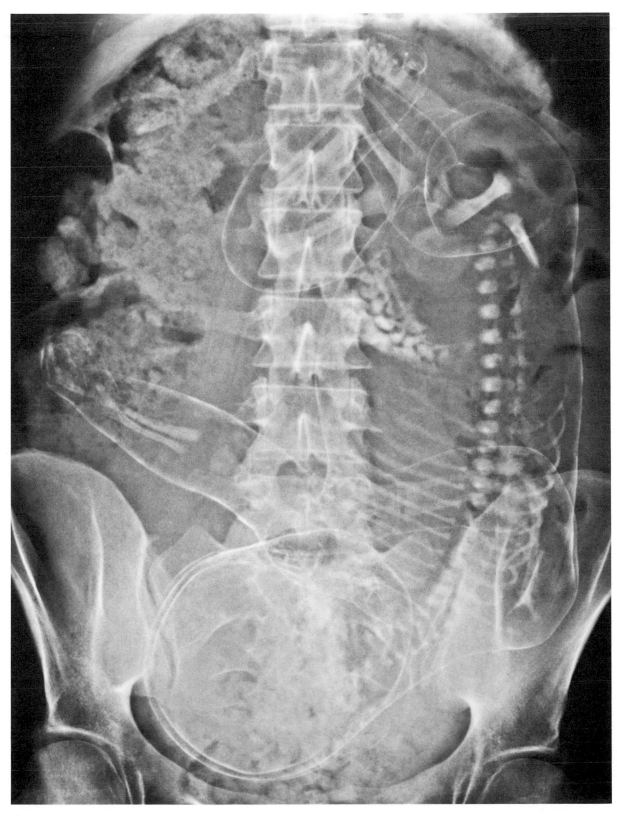

Fig. 128. Fetogram

# Bibliography

*Benninghoff-Goerttler:* Lehrbuch der Anatomie des Menschen (Bd. 1–3). Urban & Schwarzenberg, München–Berlin–Wien 1975.

*Feneis, H.:* Anatomisches Bildwörterbuch der internationalen Nomenklatur, 3. Aufl. Thieme, Stuttgart 1972.

*Goldhamer, K.:* Normale Anatomie des Kopfes im Röntgenbild. In: Radiologische Praktika, Bd. XII (1930) und Bd. XIII (1931). Thieme, Leipzig.

*Grashey, R., R. Birkner:* Atlas typischer Röntgenbilder vom normalen Menschen, Urban & Schwarzenberg, München–Berlin 1964.

*Hoxter, E. A.:* Röntgenaufnahmetechnik. Siemens AG (1972).

*Janker, R.:* Röntgenbilder. Atlas der normierten Aufnahmen. Röntgenaufnahmetechnik II, Springer, Berlin–Heidelberg–New York 1976

*Kretschmann, H.-J., M. Kaltenbach:* Anatomy and Nomenclature of Coronary Arteries. Coronary Heart Disease. Internationales Symposium in Frankfurt, 22.–24. 1. 1970. Thieme, Stuttgart 1971.

*Meschan, I.:* An Atlas of Anatomy Basic to Radiology, W. B. Saunders Company, Philadelphia–London–Toronto 1975.

*May, R., R. Nißl:* Die Phlebographie der unteren Extremität. Thieme, Stuttgart 1973.

*Mayer, E. G.:* Diagnose und Differenzialdiagnose in der Schädelröntgenologie. Springer, Wien 1959.

Nomina Anatomica, 3rd edition. Excerpta medica Foundation, Amsterdam, New York, London, Milan, Tokyo, Buenos Aires 1966.

*Simon, G.:* Principles of Chest X-Ray Diagnosis. Butterworths, London 1971.

*Taenzer, V.:* Röntgendiagnostik mit jodhaltigen Kontrastmitteln. Verlag Brüder Hartmann, Berlin 1971.

*Toldt-Hochstetter:* Anatomischer Atlas, 24. Aufl. Bd. 1 (1963), Bd. 2 und 3 (1969). Urban & Schwarzenberg, München–Berlin–Wien.

*Wenz, W.:* Abdominale Angiographie. Springer, Berlin–Heidelberg–New York 1972.

*Wicke, L., W. Firbas:* Beitrag über die arterielle Gefäßversorgung des Herzens. Herz/Kreislauf 7, Nr. 5 (1975), 256–262.

*Zdansky, E.:* Röntgendiagnostik des Herzens und der großen Gefäße. Springer, Wien 1939.

# Subject Index

Acetabular angle 94
– crest (margin) 68, 90, 94
– fossa 68, 90, 92, 94
Acetabulum 90, 92, 94
Acromion 74, 76
Alar folds 100
Angle, acetabular 94
– mandibular 2, 4, 44, 48, 50, 52, 156
– of scapula, inferior 74
– – superior 44, 74, 116, 156
– of sternum 118, 146
Ankle bone see Talus
Aorta, abdominal 72, 206
– arch of 116, 120, 132, 136, 140, 142, 164
– ascending 134, 136, 140, 142
– bulb of 140
– descending 56, 120, 132, 134, 136, 140, 142
Apex of head of fibula 96, 98
– of petrous portion of temporal bone 16
– of pyramid 16
Aqueduct, cerebral (Sylvius) 42
Arcade, colonic 180
– ileal 180
Arch of aorta 116, 120, 132, 136, 140, 142, 164
– of atlas 2, 4, 6, 46, 48
– of cricoid cartilage 158
dental, inferior 10, 12, 46
– – superior 10, 12, 46
– palmar arterial, deep 88
– – – superficial 88
– vertebral, lamina of 56, 58, 62
– – pedicle of 54, 56, 58, 62
– zygomatic 2, 6, 8, 12, 14
Artery (-ies) (-ia)
– appendicular 180
– arcuate 204
– basilar 32, 34
– brachial 80
– – deep 80
– brachiocephalic 140, 142
– calcarine 32
– callosomarginal 20, 22
– carotid, common 140, 142
– – internal 20, 22
– cerebellar inferior, anterior 34
– – – posterior 32, 34
– – superior 32, 34
– cerebral anterior 20, 22
– – middle 20, 22
– – posterior 32, 34
– – – communicating 32

Artery
– choroidal anterior 20
– – posterior 32
– – circumflex iliac, deep 72
– colic, left 182
– – middle 180
– – right 180
– collateral radial 80
– – ulnar, inferior 80
– – – superior 80
– coronary 144, 146, 148, 150
– – anterior interventricular branch 148, 150
– – – ventricular branch 144, 146, 148
– – atrioventricular node branch 144
– – circumflex branch 148, 150
– – coni arteriosi branches 144, 148
– – diagonal branch 148, 150
– – marginal branch 144, 146, 148
– – middle atrial branch 150
– – posterior atrial branch 146, 148
– – – interventricular branch 144, 146, 148
– – – ventricular branch 144, 146
– – posterolateral branch 144, 146, 148
– – septal branches 144, 148, 150
– – sinuatrial node branch 144
– cystic 176
– digital, palmar, common 88
– – – proper 88
– dorsal of foot 114
– epigastric, inferior 72
– femoral 72, 104
– – deep 72
– gastric, left 176, 206
– – right 176
– gastroduodenal 176, 206
– gastroepiploic, gastric branches 176
– – left 176
– – right 176, 206
– genicular, descending 104
– – lateral superior 104
– – medial inferior 104
– – – superior 104
– – middle 104
– gluteal superior 72
– hepatic, common 176, 206
– – left branch 176, 206
– – middle branch 176
– – proper 176, 206
– – right branch 176, 206
– ileal 180, 206
– ileocolic 180, 206
– iliac, circumflex deep 72

Artery
– – common 72, 182, 206
– – external 72
– – internal 72
– iliolumbar 72
– intercostal 142
– interosseous, anterior (volar) 80, 88
– – common 80
– – posterior (of forearm) 80
– – recurrent 80
– jejunal 180, 206
– of kidney, interlobar 204
– segmental 204
– lenticular 22
– lumbar 72, 206
– malleolar, lateral anterior 114
– mesenteric, inferior 182
– – superior 180, 206
– obturator 72
– ophthalmic 20, 22
– pancreatic, posterior 176
– pancreaticoduodenal, inferior 206
– – superior 176
– pericallosal 20, 22
– – posterior 34
– phrenic, inferior 206
– popliteal 104
– principal of thumb 88
– pudendal, internal 72
– pulmonary (left or right) 116, 120, 132, 138
– – basal part 116
– – intermediate part 116
– – lobe branches 120, 138
– radial 80, 88
– – collateral 80
– – of index finger 88
– – recurrent 80
– rectal, superior 182
– renal 204, 206
– – anterior branch 204
– – capsular branch 204
– – posterior branch 204
– – ureteric branch 204
– sacral, lateral 72
– – median 72, 206
– sigmoid 182
– splenic 176, 206
– – pancreatic branch 176
– striate, anterior (Heubner) 22
– subclavian 140, 142
– suprarenal, inferior 206
– – middle 206

*Artery*
– – superior 206
– temporal 20
– thoracic, internal 140, 142
– tibial, anterior 104, 114
– – posterior 104, 114
– ulnar 80, 88
– – collateral inferior 80
– – – superior 80
– – palmar deep branches 88
– – recurrent 80
– uterine 72
– vertebral 32, 34, 142
Articular cartilage (knee joint) 100, 102
– portion of acetabulum 68, 90, 92
Articulation(s) or Joint(s)
– acromioclavicular 74
– atlantoaxial, lateral 2, 44, 46
– atlantooccipital 2
– calcaneocuboid 108, 110, 112
– costotransverse 56
– of hip (hip joint) 68, 70, 90, 92, 94
– interphalangeal, distal 82
– – proximal 82
– intervertebral 44, 48, 50, 52, 54, 56, 58, 70
– of knee (knee joint) 96, 98, 100, 102, 104
– metacarpophalangeal 82
– radioulnar, distal 82
– – proximal 78
– sacroiliac 62, 90, 92, 174, 186, 228
– subtalar 108
– talocalcaneonavicular 108
– talocrural (ankle joint) 106, 108
– talonavicular 108, 112
– uncovertebral 44
Atlas 50, 52, 54
– arch of 2, 4, 6, 46, 48
– posterior tubercle 4
Atrium, left 134, 136, 142, 164
– right 116, 120, 132, 136, 138, 142
Auricle see Ear
Auricle of atrium, left 116, 132, 140
– – right 138
Axis (epistropheus) 46, 48, 50, 52, 54, 162
– odontoid process 2, 4, 6, 44, 46, 48
– spinous process 4

Bifurcation of trachea 116, 120
Body or Corpus
– adipose of sole 112
– of axis 46, 48
– of gallbladder 192, 194, 196
– of hyoid bone 48
– of ischium 90, 92
– of mandible 12, 44, 46
– of metacarpal bone 82
– of scapula 74, 76
– of sternum 118, 146
– of stomach 166, 168, 170
Bone(s) see Os(sa)
Border see Crest, Margin, Ridge
Branch of pubis, inferior 68, 90
– – superior 68, 90

Bronchus, intermediate 122, 124
– lobar, inferior (left and right) 118, 120, 122, 124, 126, 128
– – middle (right) 120, 122, 124
– – superior, left 120, 126, 128
– – – right 120, 122, 124, 136
– primary, left 56, 116, 118, 120, 126, 128, 134, 136
– – right 116, 118, 120, 122, 124, 134, 136
– segmental 120, 122, 124, 126, 128
Bulb, aortic 140
– duodenal 166, 168, 172, 174
– of internal jugular vein, inferior 138
– – – – superior 28
Bursa, suprapatellar 100

Calcaneus (heel bone) 108, 110, 112
Calices, renal (upper, middle, lower) 202, 204
Canal(s)
– cervical of uterus 228
– of diploic veins 4
– incisive 18
– infraorbital 12
– mandibular 18
– nasolacrimal 18
– optic 14
– of pulp 18
– pyloric 166, 168, 172
– sacral 70
– semicircular, anterior 14
Canine tooth 18
Capitulum of humerus 78
Cardia 166
Cardiovascular angle 132
Carotid siphon 20
Carpal tunnel 84
Cartilage, articular (knee joint) 100, 102
– cricoid 158
– thyroid 156
Cauda equina 64, 66
Caudate nucleus, head of 38
Cavity (see also Space)
– articular, of knee joint 100, 102
– glenoid, of scapula 74, 76
– oral 4, 158, 162
– of septum pellucidum (also fifth ventricle) 38
– subarachnoid, with denticulate ligament 64
– tympanic 8, 16
– uterine 228
Cecum 184, 186, 190
Cerebral aqueduct (aqueduct of Sylvius) 42
Clavicle (collar bone) 44, 56, 74, 76, 116, 118, 142, 156, 160, 164, 224
Clivus (Blumenbach) 4, 6, 20, 32
Coccyx 68, 70, 90, 188
Cochlea 8, 14
Colon, ascending 180, 184, 186, 190
– descending 182, 184, 186, 188, 190
– haustra 184
– sigmoid 180, 182, 184, 186, 188, 190
– transverse 184, 186, 190, 198

Commissure, posterior 42
Concha, nasal, inferior 2, 10, 12
Condyle of femur, lateral 96, 98, 100, 102
– – medial 96, 98, 100, 102
– occipital 8
– of tibia, lateral 96
– – medial 96, 102
Cone, arterial (conus arteriosus) 134, 138
Confluence of sinuses 28, 30, 36
Corpus see Body or Shaft
Crest (see also Margin, Ridge)
– acetabular 68, 90, 94
– frontal, of frontal bone 2
– iliac 60, 62, 68, 70, 72, 180, 196, 206
– intertrochanteric, of femur 68, 90, 92, 222
– occipital, internal 14
– sacral, median 70
Crista galli 2, 4, 8, 12, 14
Cuboid bone 106, 108, 110, 112
Curvature of stomach 166, 168
Dens axis (odontoid process of axis) 2, 4, 6, 44, 46, 48

Diaphragm 116, 118, 130, 132, 134, 136, 140, 142, 146, 164, 166, 168, 178
Diaphysis, femoral 94
Diploe of frontal bone 4
Disc, intervertebral 50, 52, 60, 66
Dorsum sellae (turcicae) 4, 42
Duct, common bile 196, 198, 200
– cystic 194, 196, 198, 200
– – smooth part 196
– – valvular part 196
– hepatic, common 196, 198, 200
– – left 196, 198, 200
– – right 196, 198, 200
– – – anterior branch 198
– – – posterior branch 198
– pancreatic (Wirsung) 198
– thoracic (also alimentary or chiliferous duct) 226
Duodenal bulb 166, 168, 172, 174
– cap 170
Duodenum, ascending part 168, 170, 198
– descending part 166, 168, 170, 196, 198, 200
– horizontal part (inferior) 166, 168, 170, 198
– inferior angle (flexure) 168, 170
– superior angle (flexure) 168, 172
Dural sac 66

Ear (auricle) 16, 230
Elbow 78, 79
Eminence, iliopubic 68
– intercondylar 98, 102
Epicondyles of femur 96
– of humerus 78
Epiglottis 160
Epistropheus see Axis
Esophagus 120, 160, 162, 164, 166
Ethmoidal cells 2, 4, 6, 8, 10, 12, 14

Femur (thigh bone), adductor tubercle 96
– condyles 96, 98, 100, 102

*Femur*
- diaphysis 94
- distal 96, 98, 100, 104, 210
- epicondyles 96
- fetal 230
- head 68, 90, 92, 174, 188, 222
-- ossification center 94
- proximal 92, 94
Fibula, apex of head 96, 98
- distal 106, 108, 110, 112, 114
- fetal 230
- proximal 96, 98, 100, 104
Fimbriae of uterine tube 228
Fingers 82, 86, 88
Fissure of glottis (rima glottidis) 156
- orbital, inferior 8
-- superior (anterior) lacerate foramen 2, 12
Flexure, colic, left (splenic) 170, 180, 182, 184, 186, 190
-- right (hcpatic) 180, 184, 186, 190, 192, 196
- duodenal, inferior 168, 170
-- superior 168, 172
- duodenojejunal 168, 170, 198, 200
Fold(s)
- gastric 180
- glossoepiglottic, lateral 160
Foramen (-ina)
- infraorbital 10
- intervertebral 54, 56, 60, 62, 66
- jugular 8
- lacerum 8
- magnum 4, 6, 8
- mental 18
- obturator 68, 90, 92, 228
- oval, of sphenoid bone 8, 12
- rotundum 2, 10, 12
- spinous, of sphenoid bone 6, 8, 12
Fossa, acetabular 68, 90, 92
- articular, of mandible 16
- coronoid, of humerus 78
- cranial, middle 6, 8, 12, 42
- hypophyseal 2, 4, 10, 12, 16, 40, 42
- mandibular 14
- of olecranon 78
- radial, of humerus 78
Fovea of head of femur 68
Frontal bone, diploe 4
-- orbital part 4
Fundus of gallbladder 192, 194, 196
- of stomach 116, 166, 168, 170, 178, 198
- of uterus 228

**G**all bladder 184, 192, 194, 196, 198
- body 192, 194, 196
- fundus 192, 194, 196
- neck 192, 194, 196
Gastric folds 180
Gastroepiploic vessels 176, 206
Gland, suprarenal 208
Granular pits 2
Groove (sulcus)
- for middle meningeal artery 4, 12
- for sigmoid sinus 8, 16

*Groove*
- for sphenoparietal sinus 4
- for transverse sinus 8
Growth lines 96

**H**and 82, 84, 86, 88
Haustra of colon 184
Head of caudate nucleus 38
- of femur 68, 90, 92, 174, 188, 222
-- ossification centre 94
- fetal 230
- of fibula 96, 98, 100, 104
- of humerus 74, 76, 224
- of mandible 14, 16, 42
- of radius (capitulum radii) 78
- of rib 56
- of talus 108, 110
Heel bone see Calcaneus
Hiatus, sacral 70
Hilus, renal 204
Hip bone 184
- joint 68, 70, 90, 92, 94
Hook of hamate bone 82
Horn, anterior, of lateral ventricle 38, 40
- inferior, of lateral ventricle 40
- posterior, of lateral ventricle 40
- sacral 70
Humerus, anatomical neck 74, 76
- distal 78, 80
- epicondyles 78
- fetal 230
- head 74, 76, 224
- proximal 74, 76
- surgical neck 74, 76
- trochlea 78
- tubercles 74, 76
Hyoid bone 4, 48, 50, 158, 162
Hypophyseal fossa 2, 4, 10, 16, 40, 42

**I**leum 174
Incisive tooth 18
Interalveolar septa 18
Intervertebral articulations 44, 48, 50, 52, 54, 56, 58, 70
Intestine, fetal 230
Ischium 70
- body 90, 92
Isthmus uteri 228

**J**ejunum 166, 168, 174, 198
Joint(s) see Articulation(s)

**K**idney (ren) 62, 202, 204, 208
- hilus 204
- papilla 204
- pelvis 176, 182, 202, 204, 218
Knee joint 96, 98, 100, 102, 104

**L**abyrinth, bony 16
Lamina (see also Layer, Plate)
- of cricoid cartilage 48, 158
- of thyroid cartilage 44
- of vertebral arch 56, 58
Larynx 50

Layer (see also Lamina, Plate)
- inner, of skull bones 4
- outer, of skull bones 4
Ligament, collateral tibial 102
- patellar 100
- suspensory, of mamma 152
Line, innominate 2, 10, 12
- paravertebral 56
Linea terminalis (pelvis) 174
Liver 176
Ludloff's spot 98
Lymphatic vessels (afferent and efferent) 222
Lymph nodes, axillary 224
-- brachial 224
-- iliac 214, 216, 218, 220
-- infraclavicular 224
-- inguinal, deep 222
--- superficial 214, 220
-- paraaortic 216, 218, 220
-- pectoral 224
-- supraclavicular 224

**M**alleolus, lateral 106, 108, 110, 112
- medial 106, 108, 110
Mammary papilla 152, 154
Mandible 6, 158, 160, 162
- articular fossa 16
- body 12, 44, 46
- condylar process 4, 6, 46, 48, 50, 52, 54
- coronoid process 4, 6, 10, 12, 18, 46
- head 6
- ramus 18
Mandibular angle 2, 4, 44, 48, 50, 52, 156
Manubrium, sternal 118, 130, 146, 164
Margin (see also Crest, Ridge)
- acetabular 68, 90, 94
- infraorbital, of maxilla 12, 18
- supraorbital, of orbita 2, 12, 14
Mastoid, antrum 14, 16
- cells 2, 6, 8, 14, 16
Maxilla 2, 4, 8, 18
- alveolar process 10
- zygomatic process 4
Meatus, acoustic, external 16
-- internal 6, 8, 14, 16
Meniscus, medial, of knee joint 102
Molar tooth 18
Musculus psoas major see Psoas muscle
Myelography 64, 66

**N**eck, anatomical, of humerus 74, 76
- of femur 68, 90, 92
- of gall bladder 192, 194, 196
- of radius 78
- of rib 56
- surgical, of humerus 74, 76
- of talus 108
Notch, cardiac 166
- scapular 76
- sciatic, greater 68, 70
-- lesser 70

**O**bturator, exostosis (variant) 90
- ulnar, of radius 82

# Subject Index

Occipital bone 48, 50, 52, 54
– – groove for sigmoid sinus 8
– – – for transverse sinus 8
– spur (variant) 4
Odontoid process of axis 2, 4, 6, 44, 46, 48
Olecranon 78
Ombrédanne's vertical line 94
Orbita 2, 4, 6, 8, 10, 12, 14
– suproorbital margin 2, 12, 14
Orifice, uterine, of uterine tube 228
Os(sa) or Bone(s)
– calcis see calcaneus (heel bone) 108, 110, 112
– capitate 82, 84, 86
– coccygeal (coccyx) 68, 70, 90, 188
– coxae (hip bone) 184
– cuboid 106, 108, 110, 112
– cuneiform, intermediate 108, 110, 112
– – lateral 108, 110, 112
– – medial 106, 108, 110, 112
– frontal, diploe 4
– – orbital part 4
– hamate 82, 84, 86
– – hook 82
– hyoid 4, 48, 50, 158, 162
– lunate 82, 84, 86
– metacarpal 82, 84, 86
– metatarsal 106, 110, 112
– nasal 4, 10
– navicular 106, 108, 110, 112
– occipital 48, 50, 52, 54
– pisiform 82, 84
– pubic 90
– – inferior branch 68, 90
– – superior branch 68, 90
– sacrum 60, 66, 68, 70, 184, 188, 228
– scaphoid 82, 84, 86
– sesamoid (foot) 110, 112
– – (hand) 82, 84, 86
– sphenoid, pterygoid process 6, 8, 12
– temporal, articular tubercle 14, 16, 48
– – styloid process 2, 16, 46
– trapezium 82, 84, 86
– trapezoid 82, 86
– triquetral (triangular) 82, 84, 86
– zygomatic 6, 8, 10, 12, 14, 16
– – frontal process 4, 18
– – temporal process 18
Ossification center of femur 94
– – of ilium 94
– – of ischium 94
– – of pubis 94
– – of sternum 130

Palate, hard 4, 18
– soft 4, 158
Palatine uvula 160, 162
Pancreatic arcade 176
– duct 198
Papilla(e)
– mammary 152, 154
– renal 204
Paravertebral line 56
Patella 96, 98, 100, 102, 104
Pecten ossis pubis 92

Pedicle of vertebral arch 56, 58
Petrous bone, angle of (angulus Citelli) 16
– – apex 16
– – superior border (petrous ridge) 2, 4, 10, 12, 14, 16
Phalanges digitorum manus 82
– – pedis 110
Pharynx 4, 6, 44, 48, 50, 52, 54, 156, 160, 162
– laryngeal part 44, 156, 162
– nasal part 4
– oral part 162
– piriform recess 156, 160, 162, 164
Plane, sphenoidal 2, 4, 10, 12, 14, 42
Plate (see also Lamina, Layer)
– cribriform, of ethmoid bone 4
Pleura, mediastinal 120
Pore, acoustic, external 4
Premolar tooth 18
Process, alveolar, of maxilla 10
– articular, inferior, of vertebrae 48, 56, 58, 60, 62
– – superior of vertebrae 48, 54, 56, 58, 60, 62
– clinoid, anterior 4, 8, 42
– – posterior 4, 42
– condylar, of mandible 4, 6, 46, 48, 50, 52, 54
– coracoid, of scapula 74, 76, 224
– coronoid, of mandible 4, 6, 10, 12, 18, 46
– – of ulna 78
– costal 58, 60, 62
– frontal, of zygomatic bone 4, 18
– mastoid 2, 4, 14, 16, 54
– odontoid, of axis (dens axis) 2, 4, 6, 44, 46, 48
– posterior, of talus 108, 112
– pterygoid, of sphenoid bone 6, 8, 12
– spinous 44, 48, 54, 62, 70
– styloid, of radius 82, 84
– – of temporal bone 2, 16, 46
– – of ulna 82, 84, 86
– temporal, of zygomatic bone 18
– transverse, of atlas 2, 46
– – of axis 48
– – of vertebrae 44, 48, 56
– uncinate 44, 48
– ungulate 82
– zygomatic 4
Promontory of sacrum 60, 70
Protuberance, mental 2, 4, 18, 46
Psoas muscle, contour 62, 196, 202, 208
Pubic bone 68, 90
– symphysis 68, 90, 190
Pulp of tooth 18
Pyloric antrum 166, 168, 170, 172
Pyramid 16
Radius 78, 82, 84, 86
– fetal 230
– styloid process 82, 84

Recess, costodiaphragmatic 116
– infundibular 42
– optic 42
– periradicular 64

Recess
– pineal 42
– piriform, of pharynx 156, 160, 162, 164
– suprapineal 42
Rectum 184, 186, 188, 190
– ampulla 188
– transverse fold (Kohlrausch) 188
Ren see Kidney
Retrocardiac space 130
Retrosternal space 130
Rib I 44, 54, 56, 156
Ribs I–XII 116
Ribs XI, XII 60, 62, 194, 196
Ridge (see also Crest, Margin)
– petrous 2, 4, 10, 12, 14, 16, 42
Rima glottidis 156
Root canal of tooth (pulp canal) 18

Sacrum 60, 66, 68, 70, 184, 188, 228
Scapula 74, 76, 164, 224
– angle, inferior 74
– – superior 44, 74, 116, 156
– coracoid process 74, 76, 224
– fetal 230
Septum, nasal 2, 6, 8, 10, 12, 18
– pellucid 38
Shaft of femur 92
– of fibula 96
– of humerus 76
– of tibia 96
Shenton's line 94
Sinus, aortic 150
– frontal 2, 4, 10, 12, 14, 38
– maxillary (Highmore) 2, 4, 6, 8, 10, 12, 14, 18
– occipital 28, 30
– phrenicocostalis (recess, costodiaphragmatic) 116
– sagittal, superior 24, 26, 28, 30, 36
– sigmoid 4, 28, 30
– sphenoidal 4, 6, 8, 10, 12, 14, 16, 42
– sphenoparietal 28
– straight 26, 36
– tarsal 108
– transverse (of dura mater) 28, 30
Space (see also Cavity)
– intervertebral 60
– retrocardiac 130
– retrosternal 130
Spine, iliac, anterior inferior 68, 90, 92
– – – superior 68, 90, 92
– – posterior inferior 68
– – – superior 68
– ischial 68, 70, 90, 92, 228
– nasal anterior 4, 18
– – posterior 4, 6, 8
– of scapula 74, 76
Spleen 176, 178
Sternum, angle of 118, 146
– body 118, 146
– manubrium 118, 130, 146, 164
Stomach 166, 168, 170, 180
– curvature, greater 166, 168
– – lesser 166, 168
– peristaltic contraction 166, 170

Styloid process of radius 82, 84
– – of temporal bone 2, 16, 46
– – of ulna 82, 84, 86
Sulcus see Groove
Suprarenal gland 208
Surface, popliteal 98
Suture, coronal 4
– frontozygomatic 2, 4, 18
– intermaxillary 18
– lambdoid 2, 4
– occipitomastoid 16
– sagittal 2, 8, 12
– temporozygomatic 18
Symphyseal line, Hilgenreiner's 94

Talus (ankle bone) 106, 108, 110, 112, 114
– posterior process 108, 112
Teeth 18
Temporal bone, articular tubercle 14, 16, 48
– – petrous ridge 2, 4, 10, 12, 14, 16
– – styloid process 2, 16, 46
Thigh bone see Femur
Thymus 130
Tibia, condyle, lateral 96
– – medial 96, 102
– distal 106, 108, 110, 112, 114
– fetal 230
– intercondylar tubercles 96
– proximal 96, 98, 100, 104
Tongue 48
– base of 162
Trachea 44, 50, 54, 116, 118, 120, 122, 130,
    134, 136, 156, 158, 160, 162
– bifurcation 116, 120
Trochanter, greater 68, 90, 92
– lesser 68, 90, 92
Trochlea of humerus 78
– of talus 106, 108
Trunk, brachiocephalic 140, 142
– bronchomediastinal 226
– celiac 176, 206
– of corpus callosum 38
– jugular 226
– pulmonary 116, 120, 138, 140
– subclavian 226
Tube, uterine (Falloppii) 228
– – fimbriae 228
– – uterine orifice 228

Tuber see also Tubercle, Tuberosity
– of calcaneus 108
Tubercle see also Tuber, Tuberosity
– adductor, of femur 96
– of anterior scalene muscle 56
– articular, of temporal bone 14, 16, 48
– of humerus, greater 74, 76
– – lesser 74, 76
– infraglenoid 224
– intercondylar lateral (tibia) 96
– – medial (tibia) 96
– posterior (atlas) 4
– pubic 90
– of rib 44, 56, 156
– of sella turcica 4, 42
Tuberosity see also Tuber, Tubercle
– of distal phalanx (hand) 82
– ischial 68, 90, 92
– of fifth metatarsal bone 108, 110, 112
– radial 78
– of scaphoid bone 84
– of tibia 98

Ulna 78, 82, 84, 86
– coronoid process 78
– fetal 230
– styloid process 82, 84, 86
Ureter 176, 182, 202, 204, 218
Urinary bladder 68, 182, 202
Uterus 72, 228
– cervical canal 228
– isthmus 228
Uvula, palatine 160, 162

Vallecula, epiglottic 160, 162
Valva (-es)
– aortic (semilunar) 142
– ileocecal 186
– venous 210, 212
Vein(s), anastomotic inferior (Labbé) 26
– – superior (Trolard) 24, 26, 28
– axillary 138
– azygos 120, 138
– basal (Rosenthal) 36
– brachiocephalic 138
– cava inferior 116, 132
– – superior 116, 120, 132, 138, 140, 142
– cephalic 138

Vein (s)
– cerebellar superior 28, 30
– cerebral great (Galen) 36
– – internal 36
– – superficial middle 26
– – superior (Roland) 24, 26, 28, 30, 36
– choroid 36
– communicating 210
– diploic 40
– jugular external 138
– – internal 138, 140
– pontine, middle 36
– popliteal 210
– portal 178
– pulmonary 116, 118, 120, 132, 140
– saphenous, great 210
– – lesser 210
– splenic 178
– subclavian 138, 140
– subcutaneous 210
– thyreoid ima 138
Venous angle (left) 138, 226
Ventricle of cerebrum, fourth 42
– – lateral 38, 40
– – third 40, 42
– of heart, left 116, 120, 132, 134, 136, 138,
    140
– – right 136, 138
– of larynx 158, 162
Vermiform appendix 182, 186, 190
Vertebrae, cervical 44, 48, 50, 52, 54
– fetal 230
– lumbar 58, 60, 62, 64, 66, 68, 70
– sacral 94
– thoracic 56
Vestibule of larynx 156
Vomer 4, 10

Wing of ilium 68, 230
– of sphenoid bone, great 4
– – – lesser 2, 8, 12, 14
Wisdom tooth (unerupted) 18

Y-symphysis 94

Zygomatic arch 2, 6, 8, 12, 14
– bone 4, 6, 8, 10, 12, 14, 16
– process 4, 16